Choices and Decisions in Health Care

Choices and Decisions in Health Care

Edited by Andrew Grubb

School of Law and
Centre of Medical Law and Ethics
King's College, London, UK

JOHN WILEY & SONS
Chichester · New York · Brisbane · Toronto ·
Singapore

This volume is a continuation of the King's College Studies series of volumes previously published by King Edward's Hospital Fund for London.

Other Wiley Editorial Offices

John Wiley & Sons, Inc., 605 Third Avenue,
New York, NY 10158-0012, USA

Jacaranda Wiley Ltd, G.P.O. Box 859, Brisbane,
Queensland 4001, Australia

John Wiley & Sons (Canada) Ltd, 22 Worcester Road,
Rexdale, Ontario M9W 1L1, Canada

John Wiley & Sons (SEA) Pte Ltd, 37 Jalan Pemimpin #05-04,
Block B, Union Industrial Building, Singapore 2057

British Library Cataloguing in Publication Data

A catalogue record for this book is available from the British Library

ISBN 0 471 93621

Typeset in 10/12pt Garamond by Alden Multimedia Ltd, Northampton
Printed and bound in Great Britain by Biddles Ltd, Guildford and King's Lynn

Contents

Contributors

Claire Gilbert Foster is the Sanofi Winthrop Research Fellow at the Centre of Medical Law and Ethics, King's College London.

Andrew Grubb is a Barrister, and Reader in Medical Law at the Centre of Medical Law and Ethics and the Law School, King's College London.

M. A. S. Abdel Haleem is a Senior Lecturer in Arabic and Islamic Studies at the School of Oriental and African Studies, University of London.

Margot Jefferys is Emeritus Professor of Medical Sociology, University of London and a Visiting Professor at the Centre of Medical Law and Ethics, King's College London.

Bryan Jennett CBE is Emeritus Professor of Neurosurgery, University of Glasgow.

Susan Jinnett-Sack is General Counsel of Image Engineering, Inc. in Princeton, New Jersey, United States of America and a consultant in biomedical ethics.

Ludovic Kennedy is a broadcaster, writer and author.

Michael Napier is a solicitor, joint founder of Pannone Napier, senior partner of Irwin Mitchell and the Stuart Speiser Visiting Professor of Group Litigation and Disaster Law at Nottingham Law School.

Ken Oliphant is a Lecturer in Law, King's College London.

Preface

This is the seventh volume of essays on medical law and ethics published by the Centre of Medical Law and Ethics at King's College. Like its predecessors in the series, the aim of the volume is to provide a collection of essays on a wide range of topics of interest to lawyers, philosophers, health care professionals and the general public. In keeping with the origins of the series, a number of the essays have their genesis in the Lent Lecture series organised by the Centre (Kennedy, Napier, Jennett, Haleem and Jefferys).

While maintaining the theme of diversity of coverage, the subject matter of a group of the essays does relate to one important issue for medical law and ethics, namely that of decision-making and the incompetent patient, whether child or adult (Grubb, Jinnett-Sack, Jennett and Jefferys). This area throws up in stark relief the wider question of patients' rights and the role of others (and society) in making decisions about their medical care. The right-to-die litigation in the United States personified in the *Cruzan* decision of the US Supreme Court and the ever-growing number of cases in Britain strongly indicate that there is genuine concern for the plight of the incompetent patient. These essays are especially topical given the Law Commission's current project on decision-making and adult incompetents.

The remaining essays in the volume address other areas of increasing social concern: the regulation of research on humans (Gilbert Foster); the desirability of active euthanasia for terminally ill patients (Kennedy); compensation for patients injured by pharmaceutical products (Oliphant); and compensation for negligently inflicted psychiatric injury (Napier). At the time of writing, we have recently witnessed the conviction of Dr Cox for attempting to murder a terminally-ill patient in considerable pain by using a lethal injection of potassium chloride. Further, a Bill is to be presented to Parliament sponsored by Lord Winstanley concerned with, it is believed, euthanasia and advanced directives. Finally, legal action is to be taken to resolve whether a victim of the Hillsborough disaster, Tony Bland, may be disconnected from the artificial hydration and nutrition which keeps him alive in a persistent vegetative state (PVS).

Finally (but opening the volume) there is Dr Haleem's paper. This should stimulate thought in us all because it asks us to step outside the bounds of our normal deliberations, and in doing so to cast aside some of our accepted premises and consider how a different culture with, perhaps, differing values approaches questions of medical ethics.

As ever I am grateful to those at John Wiley who have toiled so hard at producing this volume, in particular Lucy Jepson and Lesley Winchester, who tolerated more delays than the average British Rail passenger!

Andrew Grubb
Centre of Medical Law and Ethics
King's College London

Medical ethics in Islam

M. A. S. Abdel Haleem

The Qur'an, the prime authority in Islam and the fundamental source of Islamic teaching, contains references to biological facts right from the second verse that was revealed to the Prophet Muhammad which speaks of the power of God shown in the creation of man from a simple origin.[1] Such verses have been the starting point in many conferences held recently in some Muslim countries about medicine in the Qur'an and Islam in general. The Prophet also made some pronouncements on health and medicinal matters and answered questions from his followers on birth control (by coitus interruptus). Since medicine deals with the human body, life and death, it was natural that Islam, whose teachings cover all areas of life, should have its own views on this. Because of such Qur'anic and Prophetic references and in view of the importance of medical matters and medicine in the Islamic culture, all the schools of Islamic law dealt with medical matters from the earliest times. With the current Islamic revival there has been inceasing interest and discussion, resulting in conferences and seminars and a growing body of publications on Islamic medicine.

In its argumentation about the power of God to resurrect the body to a further stage of life after death, the Qur'an cites, among other things, the Divine power that creates man through his different stages of development. God says:

> O you people! If you doubt the resurrection, remember that We first created you from dust, then from a living germ, then from a tiny clinging thing, then from a lump of flesh, formed and

Choices and Decisions in Health Care. Edited by A. Grubb.

unformed, so that We might manifest Our power to you. We cause to remain in the womb whatever We please for an appointed term, then We bring you forth as infants, that you may grow up and reach your prime. Some die young and some live on to an abject old age when all that they once knew, they know no more.

Qur'an 22: 5

The Prophet's teachings include some that have a bearing on health and medicine. The following sayings, for instance, are frequently quoted by writers on Islamic medicine:[2]

He was asked, "Tell us about the medicine and precautions we take: do they avert the decree of God?" to which he answered "They are part of the decree of God".

There are two gifts from God in the use of which many people do not do themselves justice: health and free time.

Cleanse your bodies, and may God purify you all.

If you hear there is a plague in a land, do not enter it, and if it strikes while you are in a land, do not leave it.

God Almighty has not created a disease for which He has not created a cure, though some may know it and others may not.

He instructed the believers: "Seek knowledge, even unto China."

It was such statements as these which inspired the early Muslims to seek out the medical knowledge of the Greeks and others, have it translated and hold it in high esteem. It is remarkable that the Muslim biographer of classical physicians (Ibn Ab i Uṣaybiʻah (d. 1269) says of Hippocrates,[3] who, to him, belonged to a pagan culture, "He was aided by divine assistance". Christian and Jewish physicians were greatly respected and favoured by Muslim heads of State.

Translation played an increasingly important role:

Before the year 800 translations were few and scanty, but after the Greek works were received in an undreamt of degree under the Caliph Ma'moun (r. 813–33) translators were active . . . The tradition of Hippocrates only followed in the shadows of Galen . . . the Arabs were influenced from 4 sides: by the Greeks, the Syrians, the Persians and the Indians.[4]

Muslim physicians developed earlier knowledge and there appeared eminent figures in medicine and surgery. Among the most creative geniuses of medieval medicine was Ibn Sina (Avicenna) (d. 959) whose book *Al-qānūn* was printed 36 times in Europe during the fifteenth and sixteenth centuries in Latin translations:[5]

> These translations of the eleventh and twelfth centuries laid the foundations of the "Arabism" in the medicine of the West, that trend which was dominant for centuries, and was reversed only in modern times, and after long arguments. For long the rule held that he who would be a good doctor must be a good Avicennist.[6]

In the Islamic tradition there is, in addition to what physicians have said in their scientific works, another genre of writing which contributed to the discussion on medical practice and ethics. There were writings connected with the office of consumer protection (*ḥisbah*). Manuals written for the officee included, among other things, chapters on the inspection of physicians, general and orthopaedic surgeons. As one example of this we can cite the famous book on the rules of *ḥisbah* by Ibn al-Ukhūwwa (d. 1329).[7] The main areas they deal with are the qualifications, physical and moral characteristics of physicians, the equipment they should keep, their rights and duties, including confidentiality and care for the patient, physically and psychologically, and the control over the physicians by the *muḥtasib*. They emphasise that only qualified physicians should practise and should take the utmost care in their practice. They attribute to the Greeks that their kings used to appoint a famous doctor to examine physicians, and cite the following as a model for medical practice:

> A doctor should ask his patient about his complaints and the causes, he should examine the symptoms and his pulse and his urine; then he should give him a prescription of medicine and write a copy of this and hand it to the patient's family, witnessed by whoever happens to be there. On the following day, he should examine the patient and write a second prescription and on the third and fourth days and so on until the patient is either cured, or dies. If he is cured, the doctor should demand his fees, but if the patient dies, his family should go to the famous doctor, show him all the prescriptions. If he finds them sound, and that there was no negligence on the part of the physician, he will tell them. If the case is different he should say to them: "Take compensation

> for your victim from the doctor because he killed him by his bad medicine and his negligence."[8]

Islamic medical ethics are based on the text of the Qur'an and the traditions of the Prophet. Another important source is the general principles of Islamic legislation,[9] which are themselves based on the Qur'an and on what scholars have conceived as the objectives of the *Sharī'ah* (Islamic law and way of life). It has been observed that the Qur'an does not introduce its injunctions as arbitrary impositions but gives them basis and justifications in what is reasonable, good and beautiful. It does not negate the person's mind or conscience, rather it appeals to them.[10] It is useful to cite some of the principles of legislation here since in their discussion of medical matters both classical and modern scholars often cited such principles as a basis for argumentation.

The first principle defines the general objective of the *Sharī'ah* as the attainment of what is beneficial to people by protecting what is essential to them and promoting what is needed and what is commendable.[11] The essentials protected by the *Sharī'ah* have been recognised as five: the person's life, mind, religion, honour and property.

Among other principles we may cite:

> "Hardship calls for relief."
> "Harm should be removed."
> "Harm should not be removed by an equal harm."
> "Where it is inevitable, the lesser of the two harms should be done."
> "Removing the harm comes first before realising the benefit."
> "Necessity makes lawful that which is prohibited."
> "The limits of necessity should be defined precisely and not exceeded."
> "Wherever benefit lies, there lies the way of the *Sharī'ah*."

It was such rules which have enriched Islamic law, allowed it to grow, and enabled scholars in the past and present to form opinions on matters and practices that faced them in different times and environments – opinions based on recognised grounds.

In the discussions of Islamic schools of law there have often appeared different opinions which arose through different interpretations of the basic texts. There is a common saying among Muslims that "Difference (of opinion) between religious scholars is a mercy" because it generates a variety of opinions from which people can choose according to different times and circumstances.

There are ethical principles that govern the adoption of opinions as well as the moral conduct of physicians and patients alike, which are enshrined in Qur'anic and prophetic teachings:

> Keep your duty to Allah as far as you are able.
>
> (Qur'an 64: 16)

This takes into account both the absolute duty and the variable capacity of the individual to perform it. When someone came to ask the Prophet about righteousness, he said to him:

> Consult your heart: righteousness is that about which the soul feels tranquil and the heart feels tranquil, and wrongdoing is that which wavers in the soul and moves to and fro in the breast even though people again and again have given you their opinion.

On another occasion he said:

> Leave that which makes you doubt for that which does not make you doubt.[12]

Such statements recognise the authority of the conscience which the Qur'an calls "The Reproaching Soul" (Q. 75: 2), instilled by God in each individual. The Qur'an, moreover, further emphasises the individual sense of responsibility and accountability by reference to the divine judgement in the Hereafter. This is continuously present in the text of the Qur'an (where the terms for the present life and the next occur in similar frequency and in apposition to one another),[13] and in the five daily prayers of the Muslim, so that a practising Muslim is reminded at least 17 times a day that he is going to meet God, "the Master of the Day of Judgement".

We shall now deal with the opinions of Islamic scholars past and present on specific medical issues, and the grounds for such opinions, selecting three areas:

1. Controlling the generation of life: infertility, contraception, artificial insemination, test-tube babies, surrogacy and choosing the sex of the child.
2. Maintaining health: seeking treatment, blood/organ donation

and transplants.
3. Termination of life: abortion, euthanasia, switching off life-support systems.

1. Controlling the generation of life

(a) Infertility

"Marry so that you may procreate and multiply!" is one of the instructions of the Prophet to his followers. Getting married is an act of worship in Islam[14] and the delights of family life, love and affection, interdependence of husband and wife, children and grandchildren, are presented in the Qur'an as signs of the grace of Allah.[15] In Islamic law, impotence on the part of the husband is grounds for divorce, and, according to many scholars, so is his infertility.[16] Muslim scholars agree that infertility can be considered an infirmity and that either or both of the couple has the right to seek treatment.[17] Seeking treatment is, in fact, an act of obedience to the Prophet's teaching, and medicine is "part of the decree of God". All modern methods and technological advances are part of this and manifestation of the "Bounteous Lord who taught man what he knew not" (Qur'an 93: 5). In this regard, artificial insemination should be conducted within Islamic ethics, as will be discussed below. Despair of the grace of God is a mark of the unbeliever.[18] The believer has, in the Qur'an, examples of prophets praying earnestly to God to grant them offspring and their prayers being answered (Qur'an 3: 38, 21: 89–90) even when, under normal circumstances, this was thought unlikely (Qur'an 19: 9). Every human effort should be made to rectify the situation, and if in the end no improvement can be brought about, then it is the mark of a believer to accept the will of God gracefully, feeling that he is not abandoned to a sense of helplessness, loss and despair:

> No misfortune befalls except by God's will,
> Whoever believes in God, He will guide his heart.
>
> Qur'an 64: 11

> Give glad tidings to those who (in the face of misfortune) endure with patience and say "We belong to God and to Him shall we return."
>
> Qur'an 2: 156

(b) Contraception

The Prophet was asked by his Companions whether it was admissible for them to practise contraception by the method known to them at the time (*'azl*, in Arabic, meaning coitus interruptus) and he did not raise any objection to this. A. H. al-Ghazālī (d. 1111) discussed this method at some length, giving such motives as: retaining the beauty and figure of the wife by reducing the frequency of conception and childbearing; fear for her life in childbirth; fear of hardship from too many children. He stresses:[19]

> Nothing of this is forbidden. The only forbidden thing is to stop the pregnancy for fear of producing daughters as is the case with some corrupt minds.

Scholars of all Islamic schools of law have agreed, like al-Ghazālī, that there is nothing wrong with this method of contraception, some stressing that it is admissible if the wife consents to it, otherwise it is inadmissible.[20] By analogy with *'azl*, other methods of contraception which prevent the union of the sperm and the egg are approved. Indeed it was argued:

> If the intention of contraception is to obtain healthy offspring, then Islamic law not only sanctions this but urges it.[21]

(c) Sterilisation

All that we have just discussed relates to contraception for a limited time. Permanent sterilisation of either husband or wife is forbidden in Islam, except to prevent the transmission of sexual, mental or other illness which is known to be hereditary, in which case it is allowed, indeed it can be said to be required by Islamic law. Although it has the effect of thwarting the desire of some individuals to have offspring, the greater harm must be averted, and averting harm comes before securing benefit.[22]

(d) Artificial insemination and test-tube babies

Artificial insemination is permissible in Islam if the egg of the wife is fertilised by the sperm of the husband:

> There is no sin, and there should not be any sense of guilt in this; it might even lead to having a child which would give the parents happiness and foster their union and affection.[23]

But if it involves fertilising a woman with a sperm from any other man than her own husband, then it is prohibited in Islam, since procreation is conducted only through marriage. Otherwise in essence and results, if not in the form of the activity, it resembles adultery.[24] There have been several annual conferences recently in Makkah, in Saudi Arabia, which dealt with this subject, starting from 1981, and the decisions were the same, that the couple or either of them has the right to seek treatment for infertility from trustworthy, efficient doctors, under stringent conditions to ensure that no third party is involved. It must not involve "any means used for conception outside the framework of the married couple" – since that is forbidden under Islamic law.[25] Therefore there is no question of "semen banks" or artificial insemination by donor.

The subject of test-tube babies was discussed in a symposium of jurists and medical doctors held in Kuwait on 25 May 1983 which reached the conclusion that it was permissible in Islam between married couples in the duration of the marriage, involving no third party, whether through semen, ovum, fetus or surrogacy.[26]

(e) Surrogacy

Surrogacy is forbidden in Islamic law, since the procreation should be done within marriage. What is involved here is the protection of the legitimate identity which is the right of the child, of which he or she may not be deprived, even under the pretext of adoption.[27] Legitimacy in Islam entails the responsibility of maintenance and care by the father, inheritance between child and parents which is ordained by the Qur'an – parents, offspring and spouses being categories whose right to inheritance cannot be denied by any of the parties or by any human legislation. Legitimacy and the relationship between parents and children in Islam goes further than life on this earth, as good parents and children will be gathered together in Paradise.[28] Legitimacy, moreover, has implications for the degree of prohibition in marriage, and within the decorum of family relations.

There is an interesting case of surrogacy when a husband has two wives and an egg from one is fertilised by his semen and implanted in the other wife, who could not otherwise bear children. The Islamic Law Academy in Makkah allowed this in

1983 since the child would be the child of that particular father anyway, but in the following year it disallowed even this form, since it still created complications and it could not be established for certain whether the mother was the donor of the egg or the carrier of the child. The majority of scholars considered that it was the one who carried the child and gave birth to it.[29]

(f) Choosing the sex of the child

This is an emotive subject in the Qur'an since it was a habit in pre-Islamic Arabia for a father to become despondent when a daughter was born to him and some resorted to burying her alive, a practice which the Qur'an condemns in the strongest language.[30] There are some poignant poems by bedouin women lamenting their treatment by such husbands, one of them protesting: "We can only produce what has been implanted in us!"[31]

To discredit the attitude of such men, the Qur'an stresses:

> God has sovereignty over the heavens and the earth. He creates what He will, He gives daughters to whom He will and sons to whom He pleases. To some He gives both sons and daughters, and He makes infertile whom He will, Omniscient is God, and Powerful.
>
> Qur'an 42: 40–50

A symposium of Muslim scholars[32] discussed the question of choosing the sex of the child in the light of modern technological advances and whether Muslim parents could benefit from such advances to obtain a child which they would dearly love to have, and whether this goes against the Divine Will. They reached the conclusion that everything which is done by modern medicine is within the power and will of God, and within the framework of the laws and causes He installed in nature. They issued the following recommendation:

> The Symposium agreed that it is inadmissible to control the sex of the child if this is done on the level of the whole nation, but if it is done at the individual level, as an attempt to fulfil the legitimate desire of the couple for the child to be a male or female with the available medical means, there is nothing against this in Islam according to the opinion of the majority of the participants in the symposium. Others considered it inadmissible, lest it might lead to the predominance of one sex over the other.

M. Al-Ghazālī, who participated in the symposium, comments:

> The preference of male over female which we have seen among the pagan pre-Islamic Arabs appears now to be practised in genetic engineering; if we meet the whims of people in preferring males and employ modern medicine for this, what would happen? The world will come to ruin sooner or later. Instead of perfecting genetic engineering, we should first perfect the engineering of morals and customs and comprehend the Qur'anic statements: "Had the truth followed their desires, the heavens, the earth and all who dwell in them would have surely been corrupted."[33]

2. Maintaining health

(a) Living a healthy life and seeking treatment

Health is a blessing from God. The Prophet said the first thing God will say to a person in the Judgement is "Have I not given you a healthy body?" The Prophet also stressed: "Your body has a right over you"; "Your eyes have a right over you." In their daily regime Muslims have to clean different parts of their bodies many times; cleansing the mouth and teeth is particularly emphasised. In addition to obligatory bathing after intercourse and menstruation, and recommended bathing on various occasions, the Prophet stressed: "It is the right of God over every Muslim that he should have a bath every seven days." Moderation in eating is also emphasised; overburdening oneself and exposing oneself to danger is forbidden by the Prophet who, moreover, exhorts his followers:

> "Strive for what benefits you, seek help from God and do not weaken";
> "A strong believer is better and preferable in the sight of God to a weak, sickly one, though there is goodness in each of them";
> "Whoever guards himself from harm will be spared it";
> "A person with an infectious disease should not be brought among healthy ones";
> "If you hear of the plague in a land do not enter it and if it strikes while you are in a land, do not leave it."

The Qur'an states:

> Do not destroy yourselves: God is merciful to you.
>
> Qur'an 4: 30

The Prophet emphasised: "God has not created a disease for which he has not created a cure, except for old age." Thus he urged: "Seek medical treatment!"

(b) Blood and organ donation

The basic principles in this area are three: first, the human dignity in life and death. Second is the harm that might result for the donor. Third, the principle of "aiding one another to what is good and pious and not to what is evil and transgression" (Qur'an 5: 2). The first two should be viewed in relation to the principle of doing the lesser of two harms, and of obtaining benefit. Muslim scholars have agreed that it is permissible to use the organs of one human, alive or dead, to treat another, to achieve real benefit. In fact it was recognised by scholars of the classical age as a collective obligation on the community to save an individual by whatever means are not harmful to another individual. "So that if they fail in fulfilling this obligation they are liable for compensation."[34] The Qur'an states:

> . . . Whoever saves a human life, it shall be as if he had saved the life of all mankind.
>
> Qur'an 5: 32

The Prophet said:

> In their mutual affection and compassion, the faithful are like one body: if one part complains of an ailment, the other parts will rally in response with fever and sleeplessness.

The conditions laid down for donation are that the benefit is genuine and known to be certain or most likely and not just imaginary or experimental; there must be a voluntary and valid consent by the donor; it must not cause a grievous harm to the donor since saving the recipient's life is certainly not more important than saving the donor's life. All human lives are equally sacred.[35]

The Islamic Law Academy in Jeddah, in its fourth session, February 1988, discussed this whole question of donations from a living or dead person or from a fetus. They came to a decision similar to what has been stated above, stressing in particular the extent of the harm and benefit and the valid consent of the donor and prohibiting any donation of an organ which is vital to the donor, allowing transplation from a dead body on condition that the deceased had permitted it before he died or his heirs after his death, or the State authority if he is unknown or has no heirs. All this is on condition that no sale is involved. The principle of human dignity works against the sale of human organs, and in Islamic law they are not valid objects for sale. As regards payment to the donor in the form of compensation or a gift, this is open to different views.[36] What applies to organ donation applies to blood donation.

3. Termination of life

(a) Abortion

This question has been repeatedly discussed in Islamic law throughout the ages. Distinction has been made between conducting abortion before or after 120 days from conception. This was originally based on a Prophetic statement that

> the creation of a person takes place in the mother's belly for forty days in the form of seed, then he is a tiny clinging thing for a like period, then a morsel of flesh for a like period, then there is sent to him the angel who blows the breath of life into him . . .[37]

The vital date of 120 days has been seen as the beginning of obvious life which the mother would feel and which is expressed in the Prophetic statement as life being breathed into the fetus.[38] Scholars are unanimous that abortion from that time onwards is prohibited in Islam because it is an aggression against an obviously living creature and it entails the obligation of payment of compensation to the full recognised extent in Islamic law if the fetus is aborted alive. If it is aborted dead, the compensation would be less. However, if it is established that the continuation of pregnancy beyond the 120 days would inevitably lead to the death of the mother, then it becomes an obligation to abort, based on the principle of the lesser of two evils, the mother being considered more important, as she is the originator of the fetus, and because her life is already well established, with social rights and obligations.[39]

As regards abortion before 120 days, there has been a difference of opinion. Some early scholars considered it lawful as it was their belief that there is no life before that date. Others considered it unlawful or, at least, objectionable, because there is life which has the potential for full realisation. A. H. Al-Ghazālī (d. 1111),[40] observing that abortion is unlike contraception since there is an act committed against an existing creature, considered it prohibited. The prohibition increases according to the development of the stages from the moment of conception when it is an injurious act to disrupt that stage of growth; when it becomes a morsel of flesh, the crime is more heinous and when life is breathed into the fetus it becomes worse, and the worst of all is to kill the person after birth. Classical jurists have in general expressed varieties of opinions on abortion, with admissibility and prohibition depending on their views of the inviolability or otherwise of the human seed in one of three distinct states: (1) the early stage of conception, some taking this to mean within 40 days; (2) the stage of *takhalluq* (taking shape before "life is breathed into the fetus"; (3) "when life is breathed into the fetus" – when the mother begins to feel its movement – which was understood to be from 120 days after conception. During the first stage some jurists considered abortion prohibited on the ground of the inviolability and dignity of the human seed; others considered it admissible if done with good cause, otherwise it is objectionable; yet others considered it admissible without any further specification. We shall shortly see how the 40 days limit figures in modern juristic thinking. In the second stage there are still various opinions but the scale is increasingly tipped more to the side of prohibition of abortion, and in the third stage there is unanimity of opinion on prohibition except for the safety of the mother.[41]

From 120 days onwards, neither the parents nor a third person has the right to bring about abortion and, if they do, they face the religious responsibility in the hereafter, financial responsibility for compensation according to Islamic norms, plus modern legal liability.[42]

A fetus in Islam has a legal identity (even if it is incomplete), separate from that of its mother, so that if the mother commits premeditated murder and has to be executed, this sentence cannot be carried out before the birth. Indeed, the Prophet ordered stay of execution for a mother until the child was born and even then she was allowed a further period to look after it.[43]

The legal identity of the fetus, however, is not full, as it has no full separate existence, but because of its recognised identity it acquires four rights: first is the lineage; second, it is entitled to its proper share in the inheritance from close relations; third, wills can be made in its name; fourth, trusts can also be made in its name, but there can be no liabilities of any kind brought against it.[44]

We have already stated that a fetus can be aborted after 120 days for the safety of the mother. The High Council for Islamic Legal Opinions in Kuwait issued the following declaration on 29 September 1984:

> It is prohibited for a medical doctor to perform abortion on a pregnant woman who has completed 120 days after conception except to save her life from a certain danger from the pregnancy.
>
> Abortion may be done with the consent of the two parents before the completion of 40 days from conception.
>
> After 40 days and before 120, abortion may not be done except in the following two circumstances:
>
> (i) If the continuation of pregnancy would cause grievous harm to the woman which she cannot bear or would continue after birth.
> (ii) If it is certain that the foetus will be born with severe deformation, or physical or mental deficiency, neither of which can be cured.
>
> Except in urgent circumstances, abortion must be done in a government hospital.
>
> After 40 days it can only be done by a decision of three specialist doctors, one of whom, at least, must be a specialist in gynaecology and obstetrics, and the decision must be agreed to by two trustworthy Muslim doctors.[45]

A Muslim in any other land can act with a clear conscience on the basis of this decision, or any other decision from similar authorities, even if it is different, since differences between schools of religious thought in Islam are considered a mercy and no school or scholars see themselves as having a monopoly on what is right.

When prohibition is established it is not open to the parents, doctors, social workers or anyone else to violate it, and if they manage to escape legal liability in this world they are reminded in the Qur'an:

> Be mindful of the Day when you shall all be returned to God,

> when every soul shall be requited according to what it has done. None shall be wronged.
>
> Qur'an 2: 281

(b) Euthanasia

It is quite significant that in the volumes of work that have appeared on modern medical procedures in Islam, and even those that are dedicated to the beginning and end of life,[46] we find no mention at all of euthanasia. They speak of the termination of life only in the context of abortion. To them the subject of euthanasia was clearly not open for discussion. Suicide, however, has been discussed, in the past as well as in modern times. Here we find the Qur'anic injunctions: "Do not, with your own hands cast yourselves into destruction" 2: 195; "Do not destroy yourselves" 4: 29. There is a tradition of the Prophet which states that God said of someone who had committed suicide:

> My servant has forestalled me with respect to his own soul. I have forbidden him Paradise.

and there is a Prophetic statement in a powerful language, that

> whoever commits suicide by stabbing himself or taking poison ... will be seen in hell committing that act[47]

If the suicide does not die, there is a penalty to be applied to him in Islamic law, which is left to the judge's discretion. In fact the Prophet has commanded:

> Let none of you wish for death for a harm that has happened. If he must do so, he should rather pray, "Lord, keep me alive as long as life is good for me, and cause me to die when death is better for me."

and again:

> Whatever worry, grief or pain, even as little as that from a prick of a thorn, that may befall a believer, God will absolve him from some of his sins on account of it.

Naturally it is an obligation on society (which has been considered as one organic body) to relieve the person of pain. Life, however, is sacred:

> Whoever kills a human being, except as a punishment for murder or corruption done in the land, it shall be as if he had killed all mankind, and whoever saves a human life it shall be as if he had saved all mankind.
>
> Qur'an 5: 32

In addition to receiving fees for his work, a medical doctor in Islam shares in further rewards. The Prophet said:

> Whoever removes a worldly grief from a believer, God will remove from him one of the griefs of the day of judgement. Allah aids a servant as long as the servant aids his brother.

To call euthanasia voluntary does not change the position; neither does the individual have the right over his own life, nor is it open to him to give this to others, in accordance with the principle:

> When it is forbidden to perform an act, it is also forbidden to request its performance.

Terminating the life of those who have reached old age is even more abhorrent in Islamic ethical and social thinking, because they are in a weaker position. We have seen from the Qur'anic references cited at the beginning that abject old age is a natural stage of development in human life reached by some people and is worthy of protection and care just as is any earlier stage. It is part of the divine scheme. Caring, patiently, for parents when old has a particularly high priority in the Qur'an, coming second to the belief in the unity of God, which is the most fundamental belief in Islam:

> Your Lord has commanded that you worship none but Him, and do good to your parents. If either or both of them attain old age in your company, show them no sign of impatience, but speak to them kind words. Lower to them the wing of humility out of mercy and say: "Lord, have mercy on them as they took care of me when I was little!"
>
> Qur'an 17: 23

The verse ends on this final note of reminding the person of the time when he or she was weak and vulnerable as the parents are in their old age, and when they took care of him or her. We have already mentioned that the relationship between child and parent continues beyond death.

(c) Turning off life-support systems

Doctors are under the obligation to keep the life-support systems connected to a person as long as this is to protect his or her life, rather than prolong their dying. After the death of the brain, which is recognised as the proper criterion for death, it is a sign of respect for the patient and his relatives to terminate the life support. To leave the support system on in such a case is merely prolonging the process of dying and the suffering of the relatives, and is wasteful of resources, both of the relatives and of the State.[48]

Before the death of the brain a doctor may not disconnect the support system from one patient to use it for another patient in the same condition, since all people are equal and harm may not be removed by an equal harm. If the doctor has one support system and more than one patient in the same condition and has to decide to whom the system should be connected, he has only the general principle of "the greater benefit" which takes regard only of objective and social criteria; for example, a mother who has children and family to support and another person who does not. Here the benefits are equal on the individual level but different on the social level.[49]

Discussions on Islamic medical ethics have kept abreast with the most up-to-date medical research. Medical research in Islam is an obligation in accordance with the general juristic rule: "What is necessary for the realisation of something obligatory is itself obligatory."[50] Those engaged in research, physicians in the practice of their profession, have religious rewards in Islam and can only be encouraged in their work by the Prophetic statement:

> Whoever makes an effort to find a solution and fails, or goes wrong, will have one reward; if he succeeds he will have two rewards.

These are religious rewards, in addition to their financial rewards and satisfaction in their work.

In 1981 a conference on Islamic medicine was held in Kuwait to mark the beginning of the fifteenth Islamic century. More than a hundred medical doctors and scholars from various parts of the Muslim world participated, who at the end adopted the following doctor's oath and recommended it to the concerned authorities in Muslim countries for adoption:

> I swear by God, the Great, to have regard for God in the exercise of my profession, to protect human life in all its stages and under all circumstances, doing my utmost to save it from death, illness, pain and anxiety;
> To preserve people's dignity, protect their privacy and keep their secrets;
> To be, always, an instrument of God's mercy, extending my medical care to near and far, virtuous and sinner, friend and enemy;
> To strive in the pursuit of knowledge and to put it to use for the benefit but not the harm of Mankind;
> To revere my teacher, teach my junior, and be a brother to members of the Medical Profession to cooperate with them in what is good and legitimate;
> To live out my life according to my Faith, in private and in public, avoiding anything that might blemish me in the eyes of God, His apostle and my fellows in faith;
> And may God be my witness in this oath I swear.[51]

By comparison with the oath of Hippocrates, references to religious authority and sentiments are understandably manifest in this Islamic oath, which nonetheless incorporates the main elements of the venerable old oath.

In Islam, putting medicine within the religious context has only proved beneficial to it. Religious scholars have full recognition of the authority of medical doctors in their own profession; the authority of expertise in any field or area is recognised in the Qur'an.

> Ask those who have knowledge, if you do not know.
>
> Qur'an 21: 7

In addition to the legal sanctions in this world, medical practice in a religious context is protected further by the religious conscience and the sense of accountability at the Divine Judgement. The Islamic achievements in medicine in the Middle Ages showed that, far from hindering medical achievements, Islam pushed them forward to an unprecedented level. The prophetic statement that "God has not created an illness for which He has not created a cure, although some may know it and some may not" asserts the cure and will always urge those who do not know it to look for it. The Prophet and his followers are urged, in the Qur'an (20: 114), to pray:

> Lord, increase me in knowledge!

Notes and references

1. Qur'an 92: 2, see also 22: 5, 23: 12–16, 39: 6. 75: 36–40; M. Bucaille, *The Bible, the Qur'an and Science* (Indiana: American Trust Publications, 1978) at 148–207.
2. The Prophetic statements in this article are taken from the recognised books of *Ḥadīth*. Detailed citations have been given in al-'Awaḍī (ed.) *Islamic Medicine* (in Arabic) (Kuwait, 1981) at 717–21, and M. Ḥ. al-Khayyāṭ, *Health in Islamic Law* (Amman, 1987), *passim*.
3. *Biographies of Physicians* (in Arabic), I (Beirut, 1979) at 41.
4. M. Ullmann, *Islamic Medicine* (Edinburgh University Press, 1978) at 8–9, 11, 20.
5. M. Ullmann, op cit at 46.
6. Ibid at 54.
7. Published by the General Book Organization (Cairo, 1976) at 253–9.
8. Ibid at 255–6.
9. M. A. al-Zarqā has made an extensive study of many of these rules; see his *General Introduction to Islamic Law* (in Arabic) vol. 2 (Damascus, 1963) at 959 ff.
10. See M. Draz, *La morale du Quran* (Al-Azhar, Cairo, 1950).
11. A. Khallāf, *Islamic Jurisprudence* (in Arabic) (Cairo, 1977) at 197–207.
12. *An-Nawawi's Forty Hadiths*, Hadith no. 27, 11, translated by E. Ibrahim and D. Johnson-Davies (Damascus: Dar al-Qur'an, 1976) at 52, 90.
13. M. Abdel Haleem. "The hereafter and the here-and-now in the Qur'an", *Islamic Quarterly*, XXXIII, 2 (London, 1989) at 118–31.
14. M. al-Ghazālī, *Issues concerning Women* (in Arabic) (Cairo, 1990) at 108.
15. Qur'an 16: 72, 30: 21, 2: 87.
16. M. S. Madkūr, "The Islamic view of sterilization and abortion" in *Family Planning in Islam* (in Arabic) (Beirut, 1973) at 293.
17. M. A. al-Bārr, *The Ethics of Artificial Fertilization* (in Arabic) (Jeddah, 1987) at 135.
18. Qur'an 12: 87.
19. *Revival of the Religious Sciences* (in Arabic) II, 1st edn. (Beirut) at 47.
20. M. S. Madkūr, op cit at 290–1.
21. M. Shaltūt, *Legal Opinions on Diverse Matters* (in Arabic) (Cairo, 1983) at 297.
22. Madkūr, op cit at 291–2; Shaltūt, ibid at 294–7.
23. Shaltūt, op cit at 328.
24. Shaltūt, ibid at 328.
25. M. A. al-Bārr, *Ethics of Artificial Fertilization* (in Arabic) (Jeddah, 1987) at 134–8.
26. A. R. al-Jindī (ed.), *Procreation in Islam* (in Arabic) (Kuwait, 1985).
27. Qur'an 33: 4–5.
28. Qur'an 52: 21.
29. Al-Bārr, op cit at 138.

30. Qur'an 16: 58–9.
31. M. al-Ghazālī, op cit at 211.
32. M. al-Ghazālī, op cit at 213–14.
33. Qur'an 23: 71, quoted in M. al-Ghazālī, op cit at 211–14.
34. A. Sharaf al-Dīn, "Modern medical procedures and Islamic Law", in M. A. al-'Awadī (ed.) *Medicine in Islam*, vol. 1 (Kuwait, 1982) at 569–74.
35. Sharaf al-Dīn, ibid at 573.
36. H. A. Shādhilī, *Human Organ Transplants in Islamic Law* (in Arabic) (Cairo, 1989) at 183–6.
37. *Nawawi's Forty Hadiths*, op cit at 36.
38. Shaltūt, op cit at 291.
39. Shaltūt, op cit at 289–90.
40. Op cit at 47.
41. See T. Al-Wā'ī, "Abortion in Islamic law" in Al-Jindī (ed.), op cit at 166–76.
42. Ḥ. Ḥatḥūt, "On deliberate abortion", *Islam and Family Planning*, op cit at 340–6.
43. Ibid at 345.
44. M. A. al-Zarqā. *General Introduction to Islamic Law* (in Arabic), vol. 2 (Damascus, 1964) at 749–51
45. Al-'Awaḍī (ed.), op cit at 128–9.
46. A. A. al-Awaḍī, (ed.), *Human Life, its Beginning and End in Islamic Law* (in Arabic) (Kuwait: Islamic Organization of Medical Sciences, 1985).
47. Shaltūt, op cit at 421.
48. Symposium of jurists and medical doctors in Doha, Qatar; see al-Ahrám (in Arabic) (London, 1992) at 8.
49. Sharaf al-Dīn, op cit at 576–80.
50. A. Ḥasaballah, *Principles of Islamic Jurisprudence* (Cairo, 1967) at 356.
51. Al-'Awaḍī (ed.) op cit at 700.

Voluntary euthanasia

Ludovic Kennedy

Many of the views that people hold, and hold strongly, are the result of personal experience. So it was with me and the subject of voluntary euthanasia; and by voluntary euthanasia I mean one thing only: medical assistance in terminating life at the request of the patient and of no other.

When my mother was 80 she went to live in a private nursing home where I visited her regularly. She was not terminally ill in the sense of having cancer or some other fell disease, but her whole system had run down. Chronic arthritis and moments of giddiness kept her mostly in bed, and failing eyesight meant that she could no longer read or watch television with any degree of enjoyment. In short, life had become a burden to her. When she was 83 and I asked her on one of my visits how she was, her answer surprised me: "Oh, how I long to be gathered!" – the Scottish euphemism for death. On subsequent visits she repeated this wish, adding that she had had a wonderful life, but the time had now come for it to end. But there was no means of ending it, and she survived for another year in increasing discomfort before I received a telephone call in the middle of the night that her wish had at last been granted.

Whether my mother would have been ready to embrace voluntary euthanasia had it been available, I cannot say. But what I learned from her was something I had not realised before, that while to-day's world supports an increasing number of sprightly 90-year-olds, there are many other old people whose wish to die

---

Choices and Decisions in Health Care. Edited by A. Grubb.

is no less strong than the wish of young people to live. Robert Louis Stevenson had the words to express it:

> "It is not so much that death approaches as life withdraws and withers up from round about him. He has outlived his own usefulness and almost his own enjoyment; and if there is to be no recovery, if never again will he be young and strong and passionate . . . if in fact this be veritably nightfall, he will not wish for the continuance of a twilight that only strains and disappoints the eyes, but steadfastly await the perfect darkness."

Yet every year there are an increasing number of increasingly old and increasingly sick people for whom the twilight continues unbearably and whose steadfastness in awaiting the perfect darkness often falls short of what they would wish; for the prolongation of living which has been brought about by advances in medical science has also meant the prolongation of dying. For millions of people whose span of life has been extended, its quality has been diminished. Some are suffering from cancer or a wasting muscular disease; some are in acute discomfort from vomiting, diarrhoea, insomnia, bedsores, flatulence, incontinence and general exhaustion, being fed by drips in the vein or tubes through the nose and into the stomach. The law at present does not allow doctors to grant them their pleas for merciful release. The compassion we show to sick animals by putting them out of their misery, we deny to our fellow human beings.

In the old days when most people died at home, the family doctor often felt no compunction in administering a lethal drug to help a dying patient on his or her way; but now that most people die in hospitals, doctors cannot do it without the knowledge of the nursing staff and thus, because it is a criminal offence, they endanger their professional careers. The most we can expect of doctors at present is the exercise of what is called passive euthanasia, that is the withholding of some life-sustaining drug or the giving of sufficient analgesics to alleviate pain yet which can also shorten life; but the effect of opiates such as morphine and heroin is by no means certain, and death can take a dismayingly long time. In the old days too pneumonia often came to give a terminally ill patient a quiet and comparatively speedy death; but today when pneumonia sets in, it is quelled with antibiotics which will keep the patient's heart beating for a few more miserable weeks or months.

Nor is it only the patient who suffers. In hospitals there are paid staff to look after the terminally ill; but at home the job often falls on the wife or daughter or husband, having to feed and wash and nurse, often for months on end, a loved one who no longer wishes to live and whose relentless deterioration they can only helplessly watch. "Opponents of euthanasia", says Professor Glanville Williams, "are apt to take a cynical view of the desires of relatives ... but it cannot be denied that a wife who has to nurse her husband through the last stages of some terrible disease may herself be so deeply affected by the experience that her health is ruined, either mentally or physically".[1]

There is another factor to be considered. Prolonged and miserable dying, the gradual transformation of a much-loved parent or spouse or sibling from a familiar upright figure to that of a semi-corpse can mean, when death finally comes, that they are not mourned. "I had an excellent relationship with both my parents", a woman wrote to me, "but after watching the deterioration of their personalities and minds, caused by years of pain-killing and life-saving drugs, watching their suffering and coping with their irrational behaviour, I was glad when they died." Sorting through their letters, she remembered how close they had once been and felt guilty about not mourning them. "Parents should go", she said, "when they are remembered as their true selves. Parents *should* be mourned. That is the natural, healthy way."

The word euthanasia comes from the Greek *eu*, well or good, and *thanatos*, death – the good death. And who are they for whom we are demanding the right to a good death? In a word, all those thousands of people who in increasing numbers are experiencing and will continue to experience *bad* deaths. For a start those suffering from disorders which they know are steadily going to get worse, and unable because of the law to summon medical help to end their lives in peace and dignity, take steps to end it themselves – people like Arthur Koestler, the philosopher, suffering from Parkinson's disease and advanced leukaemia, who took an overdose of barbiturates; and the painter Rory McEwen, with a brain tumour, who threw himself under a train. Some of course have failed in their attempts: here is what a correspondent wrote to me recently:

"I myself went through a harrowing experience with my beloved mother's final years. To see someone you love suffering and daily

> getting worse is torture. She had very bad and very painful rheumatoid arthritis for several years before finally coming to live with us. The cortisone she was prescribed effectively destroyed her body, but death seemed as far away as ever.
>
> At last she said, 'Tonight I'm going to do it. I'm going to cut my arteries in my room.' I never felt more helpless, more grief-stricken. I lay in bed in the next room while she tried to kill herself with a pair of scissors. The horror of that night will be with me for ever.
>
> In the morning she was still alive, though she had lost a lot of blood. We sent for the doctor and, thank God, we managed to get him to give her a quick release. But all that tragedy was so unnecessary: she could so easily have been spared that final agony."

That old lady could be said to have been lucky. Another doctor, perhaps most, would have whisked her off to the hospital to be resuscitated.

Here are the words of another correspondent, a retired Metropolitan police sergeant:

> "I suffer from Buerger's disease. I have had twelve general anaesthetic operations in University College Hospital. I have had just one amputation, half of my left foot. I have gangrene in all four limbs. In winter my limbs are ice. In summer I perspire buckets. It is just a matter of time before another amputation is necessary due to the normal process of ageing. I will eventually become limbless. There is nothing the doctors can do."

Then there are those cases with which we are all familiar and reports of which appear in the newspapers with depressing regularity almost every month. I mean mercy killings where some member of the family, unable to endure their sufferings any longer, begs a son or daughter or wife or husband to end it for them. And one day, because the son or daughter or wife or husband themselves cannot bear to see such suffering in someone they love, they accede to the request, and then to add to their anguish, find themselves in court to answer a charge of murder or manslaughter. In the old days they would be sent to prison, though today they are usually bound over by a judge who, like the rest of court, is himself often reduced to tears by the tale of misery he has heard. Yet none of this need happen if only the suffering one was legally able to call on his doctor to help him or her on their way.

Now let me tell you first the good news and then the bad. The good news is that there is evidence of an increasing public awareness of what I have outlined so far, and with it an increasing world-wide belief that such unnecessary misery, for patients and relatives alike, should no longer be tolerated. Consider the recent growth of the voluntary euthanasia movement in the UK. A mass observation poll conducted in 1969 showed that just over 50% of the population were in favour of it. By 1976 this figure had risen to 69%, by 1985 to 72% and the most recent poll shows 75%. Recent polls in France and Canada have produced figures of more than 80%, while in 1988 on the BBC television programme *Reportage*, targeted at those between the ages of 16 and 26, some seven and a half thousand voted yes and some 700 voted no to the question, "Should those who are terminally ill be allowed to choose when to die?" The English Voluntary Euthanasia Society, formed in 1935 with a handful of members, now has more than 10 000. In the United States membership of the Euthanasia Educational Council grew from 600 in 1969 to 300 000 only six years later. In 1980 the World Right to Die Society was formed in California and only ten years later has 31 groups in 18 countries, and in 1991 concluded a very successful international conference in Holland.

No less significant have been the changing views of the medical profession. At one time they were as solidly against it as they were against abortion, and indeed some still are. But an NOP poll in 1987 found that 35% of general practitioners would be prepared to meet the wishes of a patient who no longer wished to live if it was made legal to do so, and a further 10% said they might. Among those are the stage and film director Dr Jonathan Miller and a surgeon specialising in cancers of the head and neck who wrote to me only recently, supporting the cause of voluntary euthanasia in the light of the suffering he has had to observe, and the wish of the worst afflicted of his patients to end it. From all of these facts and figures we would be right in thinking that euthanasia's time has come.

And now for the bad news. If, as I assert, euthanasia's time has come, why is it taking so long to find general acceptance? I can give you the answer in one word. Fear. Fear spread by the British Medical Association (BMA), who ought to know better, fear spread by the Roman Catholic Church who do not want to know better, fear and ignorance of the population as a whole. One has some sympathy with the BMA, for as they say themselves in their report on euthanasia, their whole training and indeed their ethos is to prolong life, not shorten it.[2] Yet they will not face up to the responsibility they must bear for methodologies which, while prolonging living, have also prolonged dying. Rather than accepting voluntary euthanasia, as many doctors do in Holland, as a last act of compassion and love to a dying patient who has requested it, they dodge the whole issue by pretending that *they* are being asked to decide to whom euthanasia should be administered and when – an entirely false assumption and one which of course they have little difficulty in refuting. The BMA report again refuses to face the problems by saying that it is now possible to give opiates to ease pain for weeks or months without, as they put it, killing the patient, but the report does not question what the patient's frame of mind might be during the weeks or months he or she is kept going, and indeed whether any longer wants to be kept going. Similarly with those suffering from spinal trauma, multiple sclerosis and other crippling diseases. "It is far more demanding and challenging to attempt to discover value in the terrible situation that exists", they say, "than to kill the patient." One is entitled to ask: value for whom, the patient or the doctor? If the patient can find value in his situation, well and good. But if he cannot and wishes to die, why refuse him help in doing so?

Then again, and continuing to avoid the issue, the BMA report says that one reason why so many dying patients ask to be given release is to see if they are still valued as individuals. "If these people are right in the supposition that their lives have little value", the report says, "then agreeing to kill them will confirm that belief". What the BMA does not seem to understand is that for these people life has lost its value and in their readiness to admit it, they are showing a courage in facing reality which the BMA and its supporters conspicuously lack. Note incidentally how wedded the BMA is to the word "killing", which I have always understood to be an act perpetrated against a person's will, as opposed to "aid in dying", which is what we are concerned with here.

The report puts forward two more arguments to defend its opposition to euthanasia: firstly that life is "God-given" and secondly that it is "sacred". For the first the report relies on its anti-euthanasia ally, the Church, and quotes the present Archbishop of York as seeing death as a surrender into the hands of

God – though it is hard to see why God should mind if a believer decided to surrender himself sooner rather than later. And because life is God-given, it is claimed, it is not for doctors to play at being God by shortening it: nature must be allowed to take its course. But doctors play at God and interfere with nature all the time. When they remove a tumour or transplant a kidney or perform a heart by-pass operation, they are interfering with nature; and if to lengthen life for good purpose, why not to abbreviate it for good purpose too?

The argument about life being sacred is nonsense. It is always held up as a cardinal belief of any civilised society, but throughout history it has been practised more in the breach than in the observance. Societies which engage in wars do not respect the sanctity of life. Societies which execute their transgressors and ask their doctors to declare that the transgressors are fit to be executed do not respect the sanctity of life. And societies which permit their doctors to terminate unwanted pregnancies do not respect it either; for while a fetus may not be an independent living being, nobody can deny that, like a bud or a chrysalis, it is a form of life; and it is hard to understand how doctors who can routinely bring to an end life which has barely begun can yet baulk at being asked to do so to lives which are all but over.

Nor can passive euthanasia, that is alleviating pain or discomfort by the administering or withdrawing of certain drugs, the effect of which will be to hasten death, ever be entirely satisfactory. The pioneer of voluntary euthanasia in Holland, Dr Pieter Admiraal, says that in only one or two instances, such as that of artificial ventilation, will death occur quickly. "In all the others", he says, "it can be long, many days, perhaps weeks. During that time the patient will suffer in different ways. Would anyone dare to assert that this amounts to the quick and peaceful death as desired by the patient and his family?"[3]

From an ethical point of view there are those who see a distinction between what the present Archbishop of York calls "administering a treatment however potentially lethal, and administering a drug which has no beneficial effects apart from killing the patient". But others, such as Dr Christian Barnard and Dr Joseph Fletcher, Professor of Medical Ethics at the University of Virginia, see it differently. "It is naive and superficial", writes Dr Fletcher, "to suppose that because doctors don't do anything positively to hasten a patient's death, they have thereby avoided complicity in his death. Not doing anything is doing something". In his view, the action of a doctor who gives a massive dose of morphine to relieve pain or who withholds treatment for pneumonia, both of which will result in death, is ethically no different from the action of a doctor who gives a lethal injection. When asked if there was not a line to be drawn between the two, Dr Fletcher said, "You don't draw lines. You assess needs. The issue is, what kind of death, an agonised or a peaceful one, death in personal integrity or in personal disintegration, a moral or a demoralised end to mortal life."

The second fear concerning euthanasia which I mentioned earlier is that engendered by the Roman Catholic Church and is less a fear of euthanasia itself as the fear and disapproval of God. The Pope, like the BMA, favours the word killing which, he says, in a Declaration of 1980 cannot be permitted in any circumstances, even for those who are suffering from an incurable disease or dying. "Furthermore", he goes on, "no one is permitted to ask for this act of killing, which would be a violation of the divine law." The Pope seems to forget that what he calls divine law is in fact fashioned by humans. He concludes by suggesting that suffering is good for one. "It has a special place", he says, "in God's saving plan; it is in fact a sharing in Christ's passion and a union with the redeeming sacrifice which he offered in obedience to the Father's will." To those who prefer others to do their thinking for them, that pronouncement will no doubt carry weight; but there will be some, like myself, who find it medieval in its attitude and barbaric in its cruelty.

And lastly we come to the fear of euthanasia by the population as a whole, and this of course is a very understandable fear, for it it based, as many understandable though erroneous beliefs are based, on ignorance. There are times, I must confess, when I wish we could dispense with the word euthanasia altogether. We know that it means the good death, but to thousands, perhaps millions of others, it means something altogether more sinister: the releasing of forces that may overwhelm us all so that none of us hereafter can call our destinies our own, that life will be so cheapened that there is a real danger that we may be snuffed out before our time. That fear has been prevalent ever since the first euthanasia debate was held, and while there are many who still hold it today, I do believe it is now in the process of being superseded by an even greater fear; and that is the fear of the *bad* death, that if the law is not changed we may have to face a future of degraded senility, our last days passed wired to machines, unable to control our bodily functions, all love of living gone. That state, we know, is the state of thousands of patients in hospitals not only in this country but all over the world. It is not death that people fear most today, it is dying.

There is, however, one country in the world where, for those who desire it, they do practise the good death. But before I come to say a word about that, let me raise a question which is often a subject for discussion – what to do about those patients who cannot speak for themselves – in particular, babies that are born severely malformed, and adults in irreversible comas. Because the only euthanasia that I believe in is voluntary, that is the expressed wish of the patient and of no other, the short answer is that in neither case should one be permitted to do anything. However, in both cases there are caveats. In that of the severely malformed infant modern medical techniques now often make it possible to spot the malformation in the womb and then, should the mother so wish it, to bring about an abortion. Where a malformed infant is born, doctors in the past have, again at the mother's request, taken steps by way of heavy sedation and dehydration, to see that the infant does not survive; and no doubt they will continue to do so.

The second group is that of the patient whose health has degenerated into what is known as PVS – persistent vegetative state. Once again, and as with the malformed infant, the patient is in no position to give his consent, and, therefore, in my view there can be no alternative to keeping him or her alive on a support machine, however distressing to relatives and other loved ones, and whatever the cost to the hospital in time, money and wasted resources. However, that situation can to some degree be pre-empted by all of us when we are healthy by making out what are called Advance Declarations or Living Wills. The Voluntary Euthanasia Society in the UK have prepared such an Advance Declaration, which they will send on request. It is shown overleaf.

TO MY FAMILY AND MY PHYSICIAN

This Declaration is made by me . . . .
at a time when I am of sound mind and after careful consideration.

If I am unable to take part in decisions about my medical care owing to my physical or mental incapacity and if I develop one or more of the medical conditions listed in Item Three below and two independent physicians conclude that there is no prospect of my recovery, I declare that my wishes are as follows:

1. I request that my life shall not be sustained by artificial means such as life-support systems, intravenous fluids or drugs, or by tube feeding.
2. I request that distressing symptoms caused either by the illness or by lack of food or fluid should be controlled by appropriate sedative treatment, even though such treatment may shorten my life
3. The said medical conditions are:
   (1) Severe and lasting brain damage sustained as a result of injury, including stroke, or disease
   (2) Advanced disseminated malignant disease.
   (3) Advanced degenerative disease of the nervous and/or muscular systems with severe limitations of independent mobility, and no satisfactory response to treatment.
   (4) Senile or pre-senile dementia, e.g. Alzheimer or multi-infarct type.
   (5) Other condition of comparable gravity.

*Cross out and initial any condition you do not wish to include.

I further declare that I hereby absolve my medical attendants from any civil liability arising from action taken in response to and in terms of this Declaration.

I reserve my right to revoke this Declaration at any time.

(Signed in the presence of two witnesses)

If you decide to sign such a declaration and lodge it with your doctor, as I have done, you would also be well advised to appoint a surrogate such as a solicitor or family friend with a power of attorney to ensure that if the need should ever arise, the Declaration is attended to; and you might also be wise, in case of accident, to apply for the Voluntary Euthanasia Society's green Medical

Emergency card (which I always keep in my wallet), which is a shorter version of the Advance Declaration. I would like to see copies of the Advance Declaration made available for patients in the waiting rooms of every doctor's surgery in the country. Unfortunately the Declaration does not yet have the force of law in this country, that is to say, that a doctor or hospital staff are not bound to see that its wishes are met, but I hope that the day is not far off when it will be. The situation in the United States is better than in the UK. The legislatures of 36 of the 50 States have passed Acts authorising the wishes of those who have signed Living Wills to be met, and just recently this advance was given a most welcome boost by the Supreme Court in the *Cruzan* case. The Court, for the first time in its history, was hearing on appeal the case of a person who had been in an irreversible coma for some years and whose family were seeking permission to withdraw her artificially provided nutrition and hydration on the grounds that this was the decision she would have reached, had she been in a position to make it. By the narrow margin of five votes to four the Court rejected the appeal on the grounds that they could not be certain, on the arguments presented, that that was what the girl *would* have wished. But they added a caveat to the effect that in future the wishes expressed in Living Wills should have all the support and backing of the federal law. My earnest hope – though it cannot affect more than a comparatively small number of patients – is that similar legislation be enacted in the UK.

I mentioned earlier that there is one country in the world where voluntary euthanasia is carried out successfully, and that is Holland. It is not legal in the sense that a Bill has been passed by the Dutch Parliament authorising it, but the Government has said that it will not prosecute any doctor who practices it, provided that certain safeguards are met. They are as follows:

1. There must be physical or mental suffering which the patient finds unbearable.
2. The wish to die must be sustained.
3. The decision to die must be the voluntary act, given in writing, of the patient.
4. The patient must have a clear understanding of his condition and of any other possibilities in the way of treatment open to him.
5. No other solution is acceptable to the patient.
6. The time and manner of death must not cause avoidable

misery to the patient's family, who should be kept informed of the situation at all stages.

7. The decision to give aid in dying must not be that of one doctor alone. Another doctor, who has no professional or social relationship with the first, must be consulted and give his approval.
8. Only a fully qualified doctor will prescribe the correct drugs and administer them.
9. The decision to give aid in dying and the actual administering of it must be done with the utmost care.
10. The patient need not be terminally ill (i.e. the decision could be that of a paraplegic).

If one had to name one Dutch doctor who has been in the forefront of the voluntary euthanasia movement, it is that of Dr Pieter Admiraal, senior anaesthetist of a large hospital in Delft. He has performed many acts of voluntary euthanasia, which he defines as "a deliberate life-shortening act in respect of an incurable patient, done so that a quick peaceful death ensues" and which he himself sees as "a dignified last act of medical care for a patient in his terminal phase". From the first he has always been entirely open in what he does. And he expresses his philosophy in simple terms. "Every patient has the right to ask for euthanasia. Every doctor has the right to perform it. Every doctor has the right to refuse it. But it is the patient who must make the decision."

Dr Admiraal believes in the importance of telling a patient the truth about his condition, even when it is terminal. "The attitude of a patient who is prepared to die", he says, "is totally different from that of one who nurtures a false hope of survival." "Few patients", he says, "ask for euthanasia as such, but are more likely to say to a nurse 'I don't want to go on like this'." To others, who do want to die but are reluctant to say so, he will introduce the option of euthanasia himself. "It can be of great comfort and value for many a patient", he says, "to know that the option is open to him."

When I use the phrase voluntary euthanasia, I am in fact speaking of assisted suicide. The Christian Church made suicide a sin from the earliest times so that until comparatively recently it was a criminal offence; and there were instances, I believe, though thankfully not many, of failed suicides being restored to health so that they could then be hanged by the neck until they were dead. Even today in England – though not in Scotland – it is still an offence to assist a suicide. But it was not always like this. The Stoics, in the third century before Christ, accepted suicide as a proper release from pain, grave illness or physical infirmities. And Socrates, himself a suicide, praised Aesculapius, the god of healing and medicine, for refusing to treat those with incurable diseases. "He did not want", wrote Socrates, "to lengthen out good for nothing lives." To the Romans suicide was also acceptable, for like the Greeks, dying well was as important as living well. "It makes a great difference", wrote Seneca, "whether a man is lengthening his life or his death. If the body is useless for service, why should one not free the struggling soul?" And anticipating Living Wills, he added, "Perhaps one ought to do this a little before the debt is due, lest when it falls due, he may be unable to perform the act."

With the advent of Christianity attitudes towards suicide changed. To take one's own life was regarded as usurping the prerogative of God; and suicides had their goods confiscated and their bodies, impaled with a stake, buried by the highway. Although the idea that suicide was a mortal sin lasted well into modern times, there were always those with the courage to speak in favour of it. Sir Thomas More in his *Utopia* urged that those suffering constant, excruciating pain (and there were no analgesics in those days) should be urged to escape to a better world. Montaigne, Bacon, John Donne, the Dean of St Paul's and Rousseau all approved of it, and David Hume wrote: "When life has become a burden, both courage and prudence should engage us to rid ourselves of existence." Primitive tribes such as the Bolivian Indians, the Hottentots and the Eskimos all made it possible for those who felt their time had come to be helped on their way.

So what are the changes in the law would I like to see? For a start nothing about euthanasia as such, no Bill in which the word, so alarming to so many, is even mentioned. No, something much simpler. A short amendment to the Homicide and Suicide Acts to state plainly that it will no longer be a crime for a qualified medical practitioner to assist a patient to die who has requested it, and with similar safeguards to those in Holland. I would add two further caveats: the first that, to avoid media attention, the only official to whom a doctor need report that he has helped a patient to die is the local coroner, and that an amendment be made to the

Coroners Act of 1988 to bring its proceedings in this respect into line with those of Scotland, where all proceedings are conducted in private. Should the coroner feel concern about any death, he will of course be at liberty to inform the police or the Director of Public Prosecutions. My other reservation is that I would think it undesirable for a doctor who has helped a patient to die to be permitted to receive a legacy from him or her to a greater value than say £100.

Lastly, there is the question of safeguards. Frankly I cannot believe that it is beyond the wit of man to devise adequate safeguards. I feel sure that those I have outlined here are sufficient to prevent abuse; and there may be others worth considering. But never in the history of mankind has any major human advance been made without some degree of risk. Surgeons sometimes make mistakes and accidentally end our lives; so do the pilots of aeroplanes. But that does not make us any the less ready to undergo surgery or to embark in airliners. All one can do about risks, when pushing forward the frontiers of human endeavour, is to see they are kept to a minimum. The alternative, of doing nothing and continuing to allow people to die in anguish and indignity, is to my mind no longer acceptable.

One final word. It is not only the law that has to be changed but our attitudes. What is needed is a totally new view of death, so that it is no longer a taboo subject and we are no longer afraid of it – though paradoxically this will be easier for those who have come to accept the idea of their own mortality.

It is time we listened to the poets, those whom Shelley called the unacknowledged legislators of the world, and who for centuries have been urging us to treat death not as an enemy but a friend.

"If I must die", wrote one of Shakespeare's characters, echoing the passage by Robert Louis Stevenson at the beginning of this chapter – "If I must die, I will encounter darkness as a bride. And hug it in my arms." And for those for whom the light is already draining from the sky, let it come sooner rather than later.

References

1. Williams, G., "Euthanasia legislation: a rejoinder to the non-religious objections" in A. B. Downing and B. Smoker (eds.), *Voluntary Euthanasia: Experts Debate the Right to Die* (London: Peter Owen, 1986) p. 156.

2. British Medical Association Working Party Report on Euthanasia (London: BMA, 1988).
3. Admiraal, P. V., "Active voluntary euthanasia" in A. B. Downey and B. Smoker (eds.), *Voluntary Euthanasia: Experts Debate the Right to Die* (London: Peter Owen, 1986) p. 184.

Treatment decisions: keeping it in the family

Andrew Grubb

Introduction

Over three-quarters of a century ago the distinguished American jurist, Benjamin Cardozo, while still in the New York Court of Appeals, expressed the legal and moral right of a patient as follows:[1]

> "Every human being of adult years and sound mind has a right to determine what shall be done with his own body; and a surgeon who performs an operation without his patient's consent commits an assault ..."

The legal right, borne of the moral obligation to respect individual autonomy or liberty, is now well accepted in England, such that in 1985 Lord Scarman stated in *Sidaway* v. *Bethlem Royal Hospital Governors* that:[2]

> "The right of 'self-determination', the description applied by some to what is no more and no less than the right of a patient to determine for himself whether he will or will not accept a doctor's advice ... [means that] a doctor who operates without the consent of the patient is ... guilty of the civil wrong of trespass to the person; he is also guilty of the criminal offence of assault."

Lord Scarman went on to describe a competent adult patient's right to consent to (or refuse) medical treatment as a "basic human right".[3] So obvious does this position now seem that it

Choices and Decisions in Health Care. Edited by A. Grubb.

was described by Lord Donaldson MR in *re F (mental patient: sterilisation)* as "incontestable".[4] In essence, therefore, a patient's moral and legal right to determine his or her fate rests with the patient.[5]

In this chapter I consider two questions. First, how does the law respond to the situation where a patient lacks sufficient understanding to be competent to consent to (or refuse) medical treatment? Throughout, the underlying themes will be, first, the desirability of a presumption in favour of family decision-making and, secondly, the need for residual (though nonetheless important) State involvement by way of judicial review.

Secondly, I consider the question of whether child patients who have achieved sufficient understanding should be protected from themselves when others consider their decisions regarding treatment foolish or unwise when, if they were adults, they would be left to make medical decisions for themselves free from outside intrusion by the family or the State. Does (and should) the law compromise a competent child patient's liberty out of concern for his or her best interests?

The juxtaposition of these contrasting situations highlights a conflict which is emerging in judicial reasoning. On the one hand, the courts recognise the rights of incompetent patients to make treatment decisions, though necessarily, through others. While, on the other hand, the court deprives an autonomous person of the right to decide because the court does not regard the decision as being in that person's "best interests" by manipulating the legal notion of competence, or by overt assertion that a decision of a competent child cannot be determinative of his medical care.

Family decision-making and the incompetent adult

Mental incapacity may be caused by any of a number of factors – through childhood, mental illness, mental retardation or trauma. Where this prevents a patient from understanding what is involved in their care, it is generally considered that the patient is unable to decide for himself. Clearly, therefore, where the patient cannot make the decision himself, others must, out of necessity, make it for him.[6] But who? As we shall see, the English common law contemplates three different "empowered" groups: the family, doctors and the courts.

The role of the medical profession is obviously important in determining a patient's medical treatment. Medical facts such as diagnosis and prognosis are uniquely a matter for medical judgment. However, what treatment *should* be given to a patient is, as in the case of competent patients, a matter for the patient herself and not a medical matter for the doctors. At most, a doctor should advise and, perhaps, even seek to encourage or persuade a patient to follow a particular course but no further; the choice is ultimately that of the patient. Why should it be any different if the patient is incompetent, except to the extent that someone else must act on the patient's behalf following consultation with the doctors?

I would argue that, in principle, the role of the "family" is central to medical decision-making in the case of a patient who is incompetent or of doubtful competence such that there should be a *presumption* in favour of the patient's immediate family being the proper decision-maker.[7] By immediate "family" I have in mind, in order of priority, spouses (or residential partners),[8] adult offspring, parents and adult brothers and sisters.[9]

There are, of course, a number of ways in which the law could effectuate family decision-making in respect of incompetent adults. Judicial acceptance of a common law right to act is only one. The Law Commission in its Consultation Paper, *Mentally Incapacitated Adults and Decision-Making: An Overview*,[10] in 1991 has suggested a number, such as a statutory scheme of guardianship or conservatorship as exists in many countries.[11] It may be that their work will lead to law reform in this area, perhaps in the direction of recognising the significant role that families can play in the case of incompetent adults.

Family decision-making in the United States

Until recently, even in America, there was little express judicial recognition of the family's role in medical decision-making. As one commentator has observed:[12]

> "... the practice of the physician and family deciding upon the treatment for the patient ... has been respected and not legally challenged. It has been accepted *sub silentio* by the law, there being little need to articulate in judicial precedent what was commonly done without reported or suspected abuse, appeared to work well in practice, and met with society's approval."

The "right-to-die" cases which began with the New Jersey

Supreme Court's decision in the Karen Quinlan case in 1976[13] have changed all that. These cases illustrate the role of the family in the care of incompetent adults. It is not my purpose here to examine in detail the approach of the courts in the United Stated – that has been done by others.[14] Instead, it suffices to see in a broad sweep the approach of the US courts in this regard. It is clear that, following the *Cruzan* decision of the US Supreme Court in 1990,[15] the federal constitution does not entrench the role of the family to make decisions.[16] That would, however, be far too myopic a vision of the position in the United States. By contrast, State laws do, on the whole,[17] empower families to make decisions in these cases.[18] The reasons are complex and are deep seated in the cultures of Western societies. The highly influential President's Commission in its 1983 Report on *Deciding to Forgo Life-Sustaining Treatment* identified five reasons for looking to the family:[19]

1. The family is generally most concerned about the good of the patient.
2. The family will also usually be most knowledgeable about the patient's goals, preferences, and values.
3. The family deserves recognition as an important social unit that ought to be treated, within limits, as a responsible decision-maker in matters that ultimately affect its members.
4. Especially in a society in which many other traditional forms of community have eroded, participation in a family is often an important dimension of personal fulfilment.
5. Since a protected sphere of privacy and autonomy is required for the flourishing of this interpersonal union, institutions and the state should be reluctant to intrude, particularly regarding matters that are personal and on which there is a wide range of opinion in society.

Adopting these as compelling reasons for accepting family decision-making, State courts have recognised and given effect to the role of family members because, better than anyone, they are likely to know what the incompetent individual would have wanted.[20] While it is a significant societal goal that a patient should be treated in his "best interests", it is irrational to seek to determine his "best interests" without reference to the patient's life history and values. Consequently, decisions taken solely on the basis that they are seen as "best" for the patient, arguably, are unjustifiable and maintain an air of the unreal. If you like, here beneficence requires respect for autonomy, i.e. a search for what would have been the patient's likely treatment choice. Reflecting this aim, most US courts have vested decision-making power in the most obvious group who are capable of achieving this: the patient's family.

In tandem with giving credence to the family's role, US courts have developed the "substituted judgment" test, in place of a "best interests" test, to further the right of the patient to choose through a proxy or surrogate decision-maker.[21] The Illinois Supreme Court in *In re Estate of Longeway*[22] explained the doctrine as follows:

> "Under substituted judgment, a surrogate decisionmaker attempts to establish, with as much accuracy as possible, what decision the patient would make if he were competent to do so. Employing this theory, the surrogate first tries to determine if the patient had expressed explicit intent regarding this type of medical treatment prior to becoming incompetent ... Where no clear intent exists, the patient's personal value system must guide the surrogate."

This approach works providing the patient (now incompetent) was once competent to express an intent or to have values and preferences in relation to medical care and treatment.[23] In cases of permanent incompetence, for example, where the individual has suffered life-long mental retardation[24] or is still a young child,[25] resort must be had to the "best interests" approach. Of course, the choice of one test over another in these instances is not inconsistent with vesting the power to decide in the family.[26]

In addition, a majority of US States have enacted legislation which allow an individual to appoint someone to make health care decisions for the patient when he becomes incompetent.[27] These so-called "durable power of attorney" statutes began with the Californian Durable Power of Attorney Health Care Act 1983 and permit a patient to appoint, *inter alia*, a family member.[28] Specifically, however, several States have enacted "family consent laws" which authorise statutorily designated family members to make health care decisions applying a "substituted judgment" test.[29]

Family decision-making in England

Re F In England the law does not vest a formal role in the family in the case of incompetent adult patients.[30] This is, perhaps, surprising given the fact that in England the culture of the family and its importance as a societal unit is well accepted and as endemic as in American society.[31] Instead, the House of Lords in *re F (mental patient: sterilisation)*[32] when faced with the question of who could consent to the sterilisation of a mentally handicapped adult woman conferred decision-making authority upon her medical carers.[33] The basis for assigning power to the medical profession was the common law doctrine of "necessity", which justifies action reasonably required without the need to obtain the consent of the patient.[34]

Underlying the approach of the House of Lords in *re F* is the assumption that in appropriate circumstances a doctor must have a legal justification for treating a patient who is unable to consent because treatment would otherwise always be unlawful *as no family member has legal authority to give (or withhold) consent on behalf of the patient.*[35] There was no necessity in this conclusion. Of course, in England there is no precedent for vesting decision-making power in the family, but until the recent "right to die" decisions this was also true in the United States. There, however, "medical practice (and good common sense) . . . [have been] subtly absorbed by the law".[36] In *re F* the House of Lords could have developed a legal role for the incompetent patient's family if the judges had chosen to do so. It must be remembered, after all, that the parental power to decide in relation to children has its roots firmly in the judge-made common law.[37] As the *Gillick* case[38] shows, the parental "right" in relation to a child "exists primarily to enable the parent to discharge his duty of maintenance, protection and education . . .". Why should it be any different if, as will often be the case, the child (now grown up) is caring for the parent (now seriously ill or infirmed)? The duty of a parent surely is transposed into the duty of the child. Why should it be the case that a family member (such as a spouse) who has the "care" of the incompetent adult is unable to make health care decisions on their behalf? Certainly, if they could make decisions this would reflect the practical, if not legal, reality in many instances.[39] At present, after *re F*, the family's role is legally ignored, but at least informally, as a matter of good practice, relatives are properly and routinely consulted by physicians in a *de facto* partnership.[40]

Further, in *re F* the House did not address the question of whether a decision should be made under the "substituted judgment" test but, instead, held that the doctors must act out of a concern for the "best interests" of the patient, which is to be judged according to what would be approved by a "responsible and competent body of relevant professional opinion".[41] Perhaps, this is not surprising once it was accepted that doctors and not the family should be empowered to decide. Also, on its own facts, *re F* was not a case where "substituted judgment" could be utilised. F had never been competent to make any decisions. Nevertheless, the judges did not even contemplate the possibility of any test other than "best interests". On the face of it, their reasoning is antithetical to the "substituted judgment" test since they founded their decision upon the *duty* of the doctor to "act in the best interests of his patient".[42] Out of this springs the doctor's justification for treating without consent. There is, however, no logical reason why a doctor should not be under a legal duty to act in the way the patient would have wanted, i.e. an application of the "substituted judgment" test if the patient had once been competent. If a patient were competent, a doctor's duty to act in his "best interest" would most certainly be tailored by the patient's wishes – that is the "basic human right" expressed by Lord Scarman in the *Sidaway* case. Why not, then, when the patient is incompetent if the patient's wishes, values or preferences are discernible? It is not as if English law is unfamiliar, at least historically, with the "substituted judgment" test. The "substituted judgment" test has its origins in English law in a series of nineteenth-century cases concerned with making financial decisions on behalf of incompetent individuals.[43] Further, as recently as 1991 the Court of Protection in *re C (a patient)*[44] applied a "substituted judgment" test in determining how an incompetent patient would have distributed his estate in a will and by making *inter vivos* gifts.[45]

In short, therefore, English law *could* accept the family's right to make medical decisions for adult family members who are incompetent either on the basis of a "substituted judgment", or if that is impossible in the particular case, a "best interests" test.

The problems of family decision-making There are, however, dangers and practical problems in vesting a patient's family with decision-making power. First, the patient may have no family, or the patient may be estranged from the family such that they are not interested in his treatment. In this situation, another decision-making process must be sought. Indeed, in some cases a patient's family may not be the closest to the patient. This has arisen acutely in the case of gay AIDS patients. Often, here, the patient's closest "family" is the partner and not one of the traditional family unit, from which he is often estranged. While the concept underlying family decision-making remains intact in this situation because "family is whomever the individual is most closely associated with",[46] the law would need to reflect this and give a broad scope to the traditional meaning of "family" for the concept to function appropriately.[47]

Secondly, there may be disagreement amongst the patient's family as to the care the patient would have wanted.[48] Disagreement would not necessarily be a problem if the law set a priority of decision-makers within the family but it would, of course, make judicial review more likely.

Thirdly, there is often a feeling that members of a family are abusing their position and acting, not out of the interests of the patient, but out of a concern for their own personal interests.[49] These may be financial where, in the case of a dying patient, inheritance is at stake or the cost of care is borne by the family or they may be emotional where the burden of caring for the patient will fall upon the family. The more significant the decision, for example, if it concerns life-sustaining treatment, the greater the fear of abuse because of what is at stake. Undoubtedly this influenced the majority of the US Supreme Court in the *Cruzan* case and led them to accept that the State *could* require "clear and convincing evidence" of the patient's wishes.[50] Chief Justice Rehnquist stated that:[51]

> "The choice between life and death is a deeply personal decision of obvious and overwhelming finality ... Not all incompetent patients will have loved ones available to serve as surrogate decision-makers ... A state is entitled to guard against potential abuses in such situations."

Fourthly, there is the danger that the family may make a mistake and simply misjudge the patient's wishes. In *Cruzan*, Rehnquist CJ opined that:[52]

> "there is no automatic assurance that the views of close family members will necessarily be the same as the patient's would have been had she been confronted with the prospect of her situation while competent."

For fear of this, the majority in *Cruzan* favoured the status quo:[53]

"An erroneous decision not to terminate results in the maintenance of the status quo; the possibility of subsequent developments such as advancements in medical science, the discovery of new evidence regarding the patient's intent, changes in law, or simply the unexpected death of the patient despite the administration of life-sustaining treatment, at least create the potential that a wrong decision will eventually be corrected or its impact mitigated. An erroneous decision to withdraw life-sustaining treatment, however, is not susceptible of correction."

On occasion, there may be some basis for the fear of abuse or an erroneous decision. But why should the law assume that the risk of either of these must always prevent members of a patient's family reaching decisions? It could be that these dangers have constrained the development of the English common law not to recognise family decision-making in the case of incompetent adults.

The court and judicial review Before we accept these dangers as sufficient to deprive the family members of their natural role, we should ask two questions. First, given the goal of furthering the patient's autonomy, is there a better way to effectuate the patient's wishes, values and preferences? Almost certainly, there is not. There is no reason to believe that doctors or the court are more likely to know or appreciate a patient's preferences or values. This is, arguably, uniquely something that family (in the widest sense) will appreciate.[54] The danger of an erroneous decision, on this basis, may actually be heightened if others, beyond the family, decide. Of course the danger of abuse will be lessened, but at what cost? The greater risk of error and, in the case of the court, the impracticality and cost of court hearings in every case when a decision about medical care has to be made, is a strong argument in favour of a *presumption* in favour of family decision-making.

The second question that should be asked is whether there is a process by which the dangers (if any) of family decision-making can be eliminated or, at least, minimised? The obvious mechanism is through court involvement resulting in judicial review or scrutiny of treatment decisions. In the United States, "right to die" cases come before the courts if there is any disagreement as to what should be done or whether there are any lingering doubts about the family's motives. To this end, courts have imposed procedural safeguards by requiring the involvement of some other review body such as a hospital ethics committee,[55] or that a guardian *ad litem* be appointed for the patient.[56]

Unlike the United States, hospital ethics committees are rare in England except in infertility clinics and centres[57] and should not be confused with the distinct Local Ethics Research Committees (LERCs) which approve research protocols.[58] Judicial review, however, is available and, as we shall see, has been invoked in many cases concerned with medical treatment of children. There, of course, the court exercises its inherent jurisdiction on behalf of the Crown as *parens patriae*. Provided a person with sufficient interest in the child's care invokes the court's jurisdiction, subject to some limitations, the court takes over the care of the child and will, itself, decide what treatment is in the best interests of the child.[59]

For incompetent adults, the House of Lords in *re F* held that the analogous *parens patriae* jurisdiction of the court no longer exists.[60] Its demise has been judicially lamented[61] and it may yet receive a new lease of life if the Law Commission, after its review of the law in this area, favours it.[62] For the present, however, judicial approval can be sought by seeking a declaration that a particular treatment (or withholding of treatment) would be lawful. This procedure was approved by the House of Lords in *re F*.

As the President's Commission pointed out in its 1983 Report, *Deciding to Forgo Life-Sustaining Treatment*, there are a number of possible advantages to routine judicial involvement when a patient is incompetent:[63]

> "First, the judicial process is a public one. Judges' actions are subject to scrutiny by the public, the press, and legal scholars. Second, judicial decisionmaking is (ideally at least) principled – with like cases decided alike and pains taken to develop reasoned bases for decisions. Third, the judicial process seeks impartiality by applying rules of evidence and by using disinterested decision-makers. Finally, the adversarial nature of the process seeks to render a full and fair hearing by encouraging proponents to bring evidence and to present arguments before a neutral judge."

These advantages (if that they be) do not unfortunately always materialise. For instance, wardship cases involving children are usually heard in private with the press and others excluded. Judgments are not always published.[64] Further, these cases often lack an adversarial nature, all parties, including parents, doctors and patients' representatives, agreeing on the course to be taken.[65] Of course, the dual aims of justice or impartiality and principled decision-making remain desirable.

By contrast, as Buchanan and Brock point out in their book *Deciding for Others*,[66] there are a number of practical and moral disadvantages to routinising judicial involvement:

> "Aside from the high financial costs of requiring court proceedings for all ... decisions or even only for all termination of life-support decisions for incompetents, the process would be cumbersome and slow. In addition, and perhaps most importantly of all, routine judicialization would fail to take seriously the special moral relationship that usually exists between the incompetent patient and his or her family ... the family is generally more likely to be knowledgeable of and most concerned about the patient's interests. Moreover, members of a family typically have a special responsibility for each other's welfare, a responsibility that emerges from the intimate nature of their union and long-standing patterns of cooperation. By entirely removing the decision-making process from the family and shifting it to a public form of debate among legal professionals who typically have no such special connection with the patient, the judicialization approach inappropriately denies any special role and standing to the family."

In the result, both the President's Commission[67] and Buchanan and Brock[68] rejected *routine* judicial involvement in preference for judicial review or scrutiny in appropriate cases brought before the court when the presumption in favour of family decision-making may have broken down.

Of course, we are still left with the central question of what role the court does play when a case comes before it. Is its role limited to supervising the legality of treatment decisions? In other words, is the court's function one of impartial judicial review or does the court act *de novo* in determining whether, and perhaps which, treatment the incompetent adult should receive? Further, must the court be involved in all or any decisions concerning the treatment of incompetent adults? Since the issues raised are common to the cases of incompetent adults and children, I postpone consideration of these questions until later when I discuss proxy decision-making and the treatment of incompetent children where these questions have more frequently been raised. For the present it suffices to accept that the availability of judicial review where there is disagreement about the appropriate treatment or a fear of abuse by the decision-maker should, in itself, be a sufficient safeguard to justify vesting decision-making power in the family of an incompetent adult patient.

Parents, children and the court

The incompetent child

In contrast to the position in respect of incompetent adults, family decision-making is the norm in the case of children. Parents have, as a result of nature, the task of caring for their children. Historically, the law in England recognised this fact[69] and, today, their obligations are enshrined in the Children Act 1989 as "parental responsibility".[70] They have, in the words of section 3(1), "all the rights, duties, powers, responsibilities and authority which by law a parent of a child has in relation to the child and his property".[71] It has long been accepted that included within this bundle of obligations is the "right" to decide in respect of medical treatment for a child.[72]

Most authoritatively, the traditional relationship between parents and their children was stated in *Gillick* v. *West Norfolk and Wisbech AHA*.[73] The House of Lords held that parents may consent to medical treatment required by their child when the treatment is in the child's "best interests". This power or responsibility is found in the common law and exists for the benefit of children who are vulnerable and unable to take care of themselves.[74]

Of course, parents may consent to medical treatment but this does not mean that the child will be treated. The decision to treat is, always, the doctor's based upon his reasonable judgment of the needs and medical "best interests" of the child. The doctor's judgment must be a reasonable one, or he may be in breach of his legal duty to the child patient if he does not act on the basis of the parents' consent. The result is that "choice of treatment is in some measure a joint decision of the doctors and the ... parents".[75]

Judicial review of parental decision-making

The presumption in favour of family decision-making is very strong in child cases, and the extent to which the State should intrude into the private decision-making of the family through, for example, the judicial process is controversial.[76] Undoubtedly, the courts have the means to become involved. Hence, the court exercising its inherent *parens patriae* power may consent to (or refuse consent to) medical treatment for a child.[77] When a child is already a ward of court, or is made so specifically for the purpose, medical treatment which amounts to a "serious step" in the life of the child may only be given with the court's consent.[78] Similarly, the court may determine whether a child should undergo medical treatment under section 8 of the Children Act 1989[79] by making a "specific issue" or "prohibited steps"[80] order in respect of any aspect of "parental responsibility" which includes appropriate medical treatment.[81] Here again the court acts in what it perceives to be the "best interests" of the child.[82]

The existence of these mechanisms is well known and generally accepted; the crucial question is how, and to what extent, should the courts exercise their *parens patriae* or statutory jurisdictions? There are three possible options the law could adopt:

1. *mandatory court review* of all (or particular) medical decisions;
2. *de novo* consideration of a child's "best interests" when the case is brought before the court;
3. *a legislative or prescriptive role* defining the scope of lawful decision-making, i.e. the relevant criteria of "best interests" *linked with a supervisory or review role* to ensure that any treatment decision falls within these legal criteria.

Mandatory court review The dangers of family decision-making have led some judges to require court involvement. In a number of "right to die" cases involving incompetent adults, American courts have imposed a procedure of *mandatory* judicial involvement.[83] On the whole, these cases are discredited today[84] and would be nothing but a curiosity if it were not for the fact that a number of English judges have flirted with the notion that court involvement in medical decision-making should be routine or mandatory in some circumstances.

The prospect of mandatory judicial involvement was first raised in England in *re B (a minor) (wardship: sterilisation)*,[85] a case concerned with the sterilisation of a 17-year-old mentally handicapped girl. In that case Lord Templeman stated that[86]

> "[a] court exercising wardship jurisdiction emanating from the Crown is the only authority which is empowered to authorise such

a drastic step as sterilisation after a full and informed investigation."

The legal basis for the view that the child's parents could not give a valid consent is very doubtful.[87] Further, as we have already seen, the need for judicial involvement in every case has already been doubted both on practical and moral grounds. Subsequently, in *re F* the House of Lords resiled from the position of requiring all sterilisation cases to be brought before the courts. A majority of the House of Lords interpreted Lord Templeman's remarks as only indicating that it should be *good medical practice* to bring sterilisation cases involving adult women or girls before the court for "approval".[88] In support of court involvement, Lord Brandon cited, *inter alia*, the dangers of a wrong decision being reached and of improper reasons or motives influencing the woman's family and doctors.[89] Arguably, if one leaves aside the emotional aspects of sterilising handicapped women, the perceived dangers are generally no greater here than elsewhere where medical treatment is recommended by a doctor. There is always the *potential* for error or, even, abuse whoever decides.[90] The availability of judicial review ought to suffice to protect the patient's interests. Later cases have restricted *re B* and *re F* to contraceptive sterilisations. In these cases, the judges decided that court involvement is not even desirable or good practice when the medical procedure is "medically indicated" or "therapeutic".[91] Consequently, English law *never requires* court involvement (unless the child is already a ward of court)[92] and there seems little inclination on the part of the English judiciary to encourage court involvement outside of the contraceptive sterilisation cases.

De novo review Given that not all cases involving the medical treatment of incompetent children must come before the court, when they do the courts in England have applied a "best interests" test, adopting an objective approach even if the court's view runs counter to the parents' wishes.[93] On one interpretation of these cases, the judges are acting *de novo* as judicial parents and determining what *in their view* is in the child's "best interests".

The overreaching effect of the court's jurisdiction based upon acting in the child's "best interests" has been particularly evident in a trilogy of wardship cases concerned with the treatment of handicapped and seriously ill babies:[94] *re B (a minor) (wardship:*

medical treatment);[95] *re C (a minor) (wardship: medical treatment)*;[96] *re J (a minor) (wardship: medical treatment)*.[97] As Lord Donaldson stated in *re J*:[98]

> "*The court* when exercising the parens patriae jurisdiction takes over the rights and duties of the parents, although this is not to say that the parents will be excluded from the decision-making process. Nevertheless the responsibility for the decision whether to give or to withhold consent is that of the court alone."

Hence, in *re B* the Court of Appeal authorised a life-saving operation on a newborn child suffering from Down's syndrome even though her parents had refused consent to the treatment, because the court concluded that it could not be demonstrated that the child's life was "demonstrably going to be so awful that [it] must be condemned to die".[99]

It is to be expected that in cases where the child will die unless treated, the courts are more likely to override parental decisions to refuse treatment because of the magnitude of the decision and the interests of the child which are in issue. However, the English cases go beyond life-and-death situations, extending the approach to all health decisions, for example sterilisation and abortion. In *re D (a minor) (wardship: sterilisation)*[100] Heilbron J refused her consent to a sterilisation of an 11-year-old girl even after her mother had consented, and in *re B (wardship: abortion)*[101] Hollis J consented to an abortion on a 12-year-old girl against her mother's religious objections.[102] While judicial involvement in cases where the child's life is not at stake can be forcefully criticised,[103] it remains arguable that the courts, as *parens patriae*, are acting *in what they perceive as the best interests of the child* once their jurisdiction has been triggered.

Are the judges justified in substituting their views of a child's best interests over that of the parents? Arguably they are not, and so another view of the case law is desirable if possible. This contemplates the courts carrying out two functions: one legislative and the other supervisory in nature. The court would now have a more limited role, though nonetheless an important one.

A legislative and review role Some have argued that the State should only become involved in extreme cases akin to abuse, abandonment or neglect. The argument for State and judicial restraint is most closely associated with the work of Joseph

Goldstein, Anna Freud and Albert Solnit.[104] Lord Mackay, the Lord Chancellor, explained the approach of English law in a lecture where he described the underlying philosophy of the Children Bill:[105]

> "The integrity and independence of the family is the basic building block of a free and democratic society and the need to defend it should be clearly perceivable in the law. Accordingly, unless there is evidence that a child is being or is likely to be positively harmed because of a failure in the family, the state, whether in the guise of a local authority, or a court, should not interfere."

The case law is compatible with this philosophy. Consistently with this approach, the court should perform a legislative function prescribing the outer limits of lawful decision-making. Hence, the court establishes criteria which must be given due consideration by the parents in reaching a decision as to a child's "best interests". The court, in other words, marks out "the four corners" of the decision-maker's discretion to determine.[106] So, for example, in the handicapped or seriously ill newborn cases the legislative function involves the court enunciating the criterion for decision-making, namely an assessment of the child's future quality of life.[107] The court requires that the parents ask themselves "is the child's life so intolerable that life would not be worth living?"

Secondly, the court scrutinises the parents' refusal to consent to the treatment and also the medical evidence, and then must be satisfied that the refusal is based upon an application of the court-enunciated criteria. In other words, the court must be satisfied that the parents have given due consideration to the relevant factors embodied in the legal standard set by the court.[108] Thus, the court acts in a supervisory capacity and *reviews* the decision of the parents.[109] In doing this, the court should bear in mind that questions of the child's medical condition, the available treatment options and prognoses are all medical matters. Armed with this knowledge, equally the court should bear in mind that which course is to be taken is not a medical decision but rather an assessment of what would be "best" for the child applying the court's criteria, i.e. the "four corners" of available discretion.[110]

A good example of an area where the court has performed this legislative and review function is the case law where the refusal to consent to the treatment is based upon the parents' religious views. Here, the medical evidence will almost certainly be unanimously in favour of treatment. It will be very difficult, perhaps impossible, for a judge to sit back and accept that a child should die, or suffer "avoidable harm" solely on the basis of, for instance, the parents' religious views. As the graphic comment of Justice Rutledge in the famous case of *Prince* v. *Massachusetts* makes clear:[111]

> "Parents may be free to become martyrs of themselves, but it does not follow that they are free in identical circumstances to make martyrs of their children ... "

Consequently, the federal courts in America have overridden the religious beliefs of parents and have authorised life-saving blood transfusion against the wishes of a child's parents who were Jehovah's Witnesses.[112] In cases where the medical need is strong and the parental choice is based upon religious grounds, how else can a judge (as society's representative) be expected to behave humanly? A judge's natural instincts are likely to lead him to protect a child's very existence (or prevent avoidable harm). Here, the presumption that parents act out of a concern for their child's "best interests" is undermined by a strong medical need and the court will attach less (maybe no) weight to the parents' views based upon a value (religious in this case) which society through the legal system determines *should* not outweigh the child's health interests.[113]

However, this kind of situation may be clear given the universal recognition of the relative merits of the claims of parental religious interests over the child's health interests. This will not, however, always be the case.

Thirdly, if there is a disagreement over which outcome is best for the child, the court should only overrule the parents if it is satisfied that the parents have not applied the correct criteria or, alternatively, the court must be satisfied that the parents have applied the correct legal criteria but in a manifestly absurd or unreasonable way. Suppose, for example, a parent refused life-sustaining treatment for a young child who independently had a "club foot" on the basis that the child could not become an athlete or sportsman in later life and the parents took the view that this would be an intolerable existence for the child. Reasoning of this sort (albeit less patent) arguably occurred in the Down's Syndrome baby case of *re B* and vitiated the parents' decision, where they manifestly misunderstood the minimum quality of life which would justify (in the view of society as represented by the court) non-treatment of a handicapped baby.[114]

Fourthly, if the parents do not fall at either of these last two hurdles, the determination of the child's "best interests" should be theirs alone. Hence, in a case (such as inoperable cancer) where treatment (or non-treatment) options both entail the chance of benefit to the child but also contemplate dangers such as pain or detriment to the child's quality of life, this assessment must be accepted as a judgment for the parents. Here, there is no "right" or "wrong" decision, merely a judgment as to the better course to take. In matters of judgment (based upon proper criteria) the court should not claim to be able to form a *better view* than the parents themselves.[115]

The competent child: re R

What role do the parents and the court play if a child is competent to make the decision herself? The need for family decision-making in the case of adults arises when individuals are unable through mental impairment to decide for themselves. Similarly, the need for court review is only justified when the family is deciding for the individual (whether adult or child) because of the dangers of proxy decision-making. Court review is not necessary, nor justified, in treatment decisions concerning a *competent* adult. The law ought to adopt the same approach when the patient is a competent child. What in law amounts to capacity to consent to treatment (competence) is, therefore, crucial.

The House of Lords in the *Gillick* case accepted that a child who has sufficient understanding of what is involved in a medical procedure (and, of course, the consequences if it is not performed) may validly consent to that medical procedure.[116] The House of Lords emphatically rejected the view that competence was attained along with a particular status, for example, reaching a certain age or adulthood. Conversely, competence, once gained, will not necessarily be lost when a particular status is attained, for example, mental illness or retirement. Instead, competence to consent i.e. understanding, was seen by the House of Lords as an aspect of intellectual and emotional maturity.[117] The "understanding" approach to capacity to make decisions is widely accepted in English law outside medical cases,[118] for example, when contracting a marriage,[119] in making a will[120] or an *inter vivos* gift[121] or when giving evidence in court.[122] Two matters are clear. First, competence is not, strictly speaking, a matter of "reasonableness" or "rationality" of decision-making.[123] Secondly, the central (and only) issue is whether the patient understands the *particular* treatment proposed. Competence or incompetence is not, in principle, an absolute state but, instead, relates to the particular decision or transaction.[124] The seriousness of the issue to be decided and the complexity of the factors relating to it will affect decision-making capacity since a person may have the capacity to understand (and therefore consent to) some matters but not others.[125]

On the face of it, therefore, after *Gillick* once a child is competent to consent (in the sense outlined above) the power of the parents (and, perhaps, the court) to consent to treatment on his behalf ceases. Their powers only exist *because he is unable to consent for himself*. The decision of the Court of Appeal in *re R (a minor: medical treatment)*[126] challenges these premisses. The court extended the notion of the court acting in a child's "best interests" to cases where the child was competent and had refused treatment.

R was a 15-year-old girl with a history of family problems. She was received into voluntary care, where her mental health deteriorated. She suffered from visual and auditory hallucinations. Her behaviour was disturbed and on occasions she became suicidal. After her mother removed her from the children's home, her condition was such that the local authority obtained an interim care order and placed her in a children's home. She became increasingly disturbed and absconded, causing serious damage to her parents' home and physically attacking them. As a consequence, an application was made under section 2 of the Mental Health Act 1983 and she was placed in an adolescent psychiatric unit. There she was sedated from time to time with her consent because she was behaving in a paranoid and hostile manner. Her mental state fluctuated between lucid rational periods and "florid psychotic" states. During the lucid periods she refused consent for the administration of drugs. The unit sought the local authority's permission to use anti-psychotic drugs but it was refused on the basis that R was lucid and not sufficiently disturbed that the Mental Health Act 1983 was applicable. The unit was not prepared to allow her to stay unless they could administer the drugs and the local authority made the girl a ward of court, asking the court to consent to the administration of medication, including anti-psychotic drugs, to control her behaviour.

The trial judge (Waite J) held that R was incompetent and authorised the treatment in her best interests. On appeal to the Court of Appeal three questions arose:

- Was R incompetent to make a decision and, if so, should the court authorise the treatment in her best interests?
- If R was competent could a parent or other acting *in loco parentis* (such as a local authority) authorise treatment against her wishes?
- If R was competent, could the court exercise its wardship jurisdiction to override her wishes?

Was R incompetent? The Court of Appeal unanimously held that R was incompetent to decide on her medical treatment and that the medication was in her "best interests". The latter is undeniable once the former conclusion has been reached. It is the conclusion that R was incompetent which is highly contentious. Lord Donaldson MR approached the question in two ways. First he doubted whether, applying the *Gillick* case, R understood sufficiently to give a valid consent or refusal of treatment. A child psychiatrist had given evidence that "[R] is mature enough to understand the nature of the proposal . . . she was rational and . . . of sufficient understanding to be able to make a decision in her own right".[127] Lord Donaldson dismissed this statement as not speaking to whether she "fully" understood not only what was to be done as treatment but also *the implications of treatment being withheld*. Since she did not seem to have been tested on the latter, there was insufficient evidence that she was competent.[128].

This is a most unsatisfactory way to deal with the case and only Lord Donaldson chose this route of narrowly interpreting the evidence. In fact, on the evidence, there was some suggestion that R was incompetent because she seems to have denied that she had suffered from hallucinations and voices and that she required medication. A person who does not accept that there is anything wrong with them, by definition, does not "fully understand" what is proposed and is incompetent.[129]

The second way in which Lord Donaldson reached the conclusion that R was incompetent was to reject the *Gillick* test of competence. This he regarded as only applicable where "what is really being looked at is an assessment of mental and emotional age, as contrasted with chronological age, but ... this test needs to be modified in the case of fluctuating mental disability to take account of that misfortune".[130]

So if we assume that on this view R passed the *Gillick* test on some days but not on others, on what basis did the court determine she was incompetent? There is little indication because Lord Donaldson offered no further guidance. Equally, Farquaharson LJ was content to state that the court had to consider "the whole of the medical background of the case as well as the doctor's opinion of the effect of its decision upon the patient's mental state".[131] He concluded that the *Gillick* test could not apply where[132]

> "the understanding and capacity of the child varies from day to day according to the effect of her illness. I would reject the application of the *Gillick* test to an on/off situation of that kind."

Staughton LJ simply agreed with the trial judge that R was incompetent.[133]

In fact, the court offered no guidance for future cases other than to say that *Gillick* did not apply. Perhaps on reflection this is explicable on the basis that once the *Gillick* test of understanding is jettisoned, the only rational basis for the court's decision can be that R was mentally disordered and such a condition is, without more, a state of legal incompetence. Such a conclusion should not go unchallenged because it is simply wrong and flies in the face of received wisdom.[134]

First, it is inconsistent with other cases where the legal competence of mental patients has arisen. So, for example, in *Mason* v. *Mason*[135] the court approached the issue of whether a mental patient could validly consent to a divorce decree on the basis of whether he could understand its nature and effect. Similarly, it is inconsistent with the cases dealing with the validity of contracts (other than for necessaries) made by mentally disordered persons that look to the understanding of the contractor.[136] If a fluctuating mental condition is, *ipso facto*, inconsistent with competence, how does this square with the contractual rule that a contract made by a person whilst unable to understand, becomes binding if subsequently ratified by him during a lucid interval?[137]

Secondly, to consider all mentally disordered persons incompetent and so unable to make any decisions about their medical treatment is inconsistent with the Mental Health Act 1983. Part IV of the Act deals with treatment of mentally disordered patients for their mental disorder.[138] It expressly recognises that mentally ill or disordered persons may be competent to make medical decisions. By virtue of section 57, psychosurgery or the surgical implantation of hormones for the purpose of reducing male sex drive[139] cannot be carried out, *inter alia* unless the patient consents, i.e. it is certified that he is "capable of understanding the nature, purpose and likely effects of the treatment".[140] Further, as a result of section 58 of the Act one basis for giving electro-convulsive therapy (ECT)[141] or administering medicines for more than three months is that the patient consents, i.e. again that he understands as we saw for section 57 treatments. Finally, it is clear from the Code of Practice issued by the Department of Health in May 1990[142] that a mentally disordered person may have the capacity to consent to medical treatment. This is spelt out in paragraphs 15.10 and 15.15 of the Code of Practice; the latter reminds us that "capacity in an individual with a mental disorder can be variable over time".

The Court of Appeal's decision not to apply "*Gillick* competence" to a mentally disordered person is doubtful and raises a number of further problems. Would the doctors have considered R incompetent if she had consented to the administration of drugs? Probably not, and yet, logically of course competence does not depend upon whether the decision is to consent to or refuse treatment. In fact, R earlier consented to treatment and no question of her competence seems to have arisen until she changed her mind. Also, if R was incompetent because of her mental condition of phasing in and out of lucidity then patients who suffer from senile dementia and suffer similar swings in lucidity are also incompetent. Does this mean that such individuals could not, for example, make a valid will during a lucid period, or if they are ever introduced, a "living will" in respect of their future medical treatment? The answer is obvious if *re R* is correct and casts even further doubt on the court's reasoning.

Finally, it is unclear why in *re R* the unit was unwilling to use the provisions of the Mental Health Act 1983, which confer powers compulsorily to admit[143] and treat patients suffering from a mental disorder without consent in certain circumstances.[144] On the face of it, R fulfilled the requirements of the Act, in essence, that she was suffering from a mental disorder of a nature which made it appropriate to receive medical treatment in hospital which was necessary for her health (or the protection of others).[145] Consent would have been irrelevant for the treatment under consideration, at least for the first three months of its administration.[146] Thereafter, R's consent could have been dispensed with if a second statutory opinion was obtained under section 58 that there was a "likelihood of its alleviating a deterioration of [R's] condition".[147]

Parents and children The *Gillick* decision has been widely understood as transferring from parents to child the power to make medical decisions once the child has reached a state in its development where she is able to understand what is involved in the relevant medical procedure, i.e. the child is competent.[148] At this point, the child (and not the parents) can consent to (or refuse) medical treatment. The *Gillick* case has been widely acclaimed as enfranchising mature children and recognising their decision-making right.[149] Speaking in the Australian High Court and relying on *Gillick* McHugh J stated:[150]

> "... the parent's authority is at an end when the child gains sufficient intellectual and emotional maturity to make an informed decision on the matter in question."

A "best interests" basis for acting can no longer, in general, be justified once an individual (whether adult or child) has achieved sufficient understanding to be competent to make a decision for themselves. At this point, the practical need for family decision-making breaks down to the extent that the competent person (here the child) can, if he wishes, act alone without family involvement because he is able to do so. The legal basis for family decision-making also disappears at the point when the individual is able to make decisions for himself. Other family members only become involved to the extent that the competent person wishes it.[151] Of course, in the vast majority of situations, the competent child will involve the parents. The point here is different: does the law elevate this *de facto* involvement to a legal right.

In *re R* it was argued that, on the assumption that R was competent, the court could not consent to treatment in the face of R's refusal if the parents could not. Only Lord Donaldson addressed this point. As we shall see, the other judges considered that the court had power to intervene and so it was unnecessary to consider the scope of the parents' powers. Lord Donaldson's *obiter* remarks are, nevertheless, significant, and given their nature call for careful analysis lest they should in the future become accepted uncritically.[152]

Lord Donaldson considered that the parents did have a legal right to consent on behalf of a competent child. Lord Donaldson stated that a competent child under 16 (by virtue of *Gillick*) or one who has reached the age of 16 (by virtue of section 8 of the Family Law Reform Act 1969) may, in law, consent to medical treatment. However, a competent child does not have, in law, the ability to veto treatment because the parents (jointly and severally) have the power to consent to the treatment and so they can override the child's refusal.[153] Of course, he pointed out that the child's refusal would be a "very important factor in the doctor's decision whether or not to treat"[154] but a doctor would act lawfully, in the sense that no battery would be committed, if he acted on the basis of the parents' consent. The court is only concerned with the *legality* of treatment and not with whether it will be carried out, that is a matter for the doctor's clinical judgment.[155]

In reaching this view, Lord Donaldson developed his argument against the heterodoxy on three fronts: (i) the *Gillick* decision itself; (ii) section 8 of the Family Law Reform Act 1969; and (iii) the practical problems a doctor would otherwise face.

(i) GILLICK Lord Donaldson considered that the House of Lords in *Gillick* was only concerned with the question of whether a competent child could consent to medical treatment in the face of parental objection or refusal of consent and the House of Lords held that he or she could. By contrast, *Gillick* was not concerned, in Lord Donaldson's view, with the distinct question of whether the parents (or one of them) could validly consent to medical treatment in the face of a competent child's refusal.[156] Lord Donaldson considered that parents and the child have concurrent power to consent and a doctor would act lawfully if he treated a child on the basis of the parents' consent alone.

This is a remarkably narrow reading of the *Gillick* decision. Of course, on its facts Lord Donaldson is correct that the case concerned only the question of a child's power to consent in the face of parental refusal. The House of Lords seems to have stated a general approach in determining the legal interrelationship of parents and children in medical decision-making. In fact, Lord Scarman's speech, both in its substance and its grand sweep, is only consistent with this wider view. Instead, Lord Donaldson indulged in a linguistic, and probably untenable, analysis of Lord Scarman's words. The relevant passage from Lord Scarman's speech is as follows:[157]

> "... as a matter of law the parental right to determine whether or not their minor child below the age of 16 will have medical treatment terminates if and when the child achieves sufficient understanding and intelligence to enable him or her to understand fully what is proposed."

Lord Donaldson interpreted Lord Scarman as being concerned to negate any parental right "to determine" whether the child should have medical treatment and he accepted that Lord Scarman (and the House in *Gillick*) had rejected the notion that the parents had a "right to determine". But, he considered that Lord Scarman intended to go no further. Lord Donaldson's view justifies being set out *in extenso*:[158]

> "A right of determination is wider than a right to consent. The parents can only have a right of determination if *either* the child has no right to consent ... or the parents ... [can] ... nullify the child's consent ... In the case in which the 'Gillick competent' child refuses treatment, but the parents consent, that consent *enables* treatment to be undertaken lawfully, but in no way determines that the child shall be so treated. In a case in which the positions are reversed, it is the child's consent which is the enabling factor and again the parents' refusal of consent is not determinative."

What, if anything is wrong with this analysis? Undoubtedly, Lord Donaldson is correct to state that the consent of the child or the consent of the parents is not determinative in the sense that, as we have already seen, a doctor still retains a clinical discretion to *determine* whether the child should receive the treatment.[159] But, it is disingenuous to interpret the *Gillick* decision and, in particular, the speech of Lord Scarman as seeking to deal with this rather limited, and frankly obvious, point.[160] The House was concerned with (and only with) the legally "enabling" (to use Lord Donaldson's word) issue of whose consent a doctor has to seek before he may treat a child, assuming that in his clinical judgment treatment is in the child's best interests. It has to be said that there are comments in *Gillick* which might support the view that the House was concerned only with the parents' right of veto, but they are not in Lord Scarman's speech.[161] Even on a literal linguistic analysis, Lord Donaldson misunderstands Lord Scarman's statement. Otherwise, the following italicised words from Lord Scarman's speech, that "the parental right to determine whether *or not*" the child will have medical treatment terminates once the child is competent, would be meaningless. Indeed, in *re R*, Staughton LJ said as much.[162] In the end, both legally and morally, consent or refusal of consent by a competent child must be opposite sides of the same coin.

(ii) SECTION 8 OF THE FAMILY LAW REFORM ACT 1969 A further argument used by Lord Donaldson to bolster his view was based upon section 8 of the Family Law Reform Act 1969. Section 8 deals with the child who has reached the age of 16 but Lord Donaldson thought that this also shed light on the position of the child under 16. Section 8(1) permits a child who has reached the age of 16 to consent to "surgical, medical or dental treatment" to the same extent as an adult, i.e. in practice there is a presumption of competence to consent. Further, section 8(1) goes on to state that in such a case "it shall not be necessary to obtain a consent from his parent". Why, Lord Donaldson asked, if the parent has no power to consent because the child is competent, does section 8(1) say it will "not be necessary" to seek the parents' consent? If the parents have no power to make decisions, not only would it not be necessary to seek their consent, but also any consent from them would be legally impossible and ineffective. They must, therefore, have the power to consent to treatment when the proviso does not apply, i.e. when the child refuses treatment. If the parents of a 16-year-old child could consent to treatment in the face of a refusal, Lord Donaldson saw no reason why this should not be the legal position for the child under 16.

But Lord Donaldson's interpretation of section 8 is surely wrong and he reads too much into it.[163] He ignores the fact that in 1969, when section 8 was enacted, it was unclear how the law apportioned responsibilities and decision-making in relation to competent children.[164] That, after all, was the era of "parental rights". It was only in 1985, because of the *Gillick* case, that the common law unequivocally recognised the child's right to decide. It is not section 8 which should condition our understanding of

Gillick, rather the reverse. With hindsight, section 8 (including the proviso) can only be explained on the basis that Parliament enacted it for the avoidance of doubt.[165] It does not justify Lord Donaldson's view of a parental right to override a competent child's refusal of treatment.

(iii) DOCTOR'S DILEMMA? Lord Donaldson's final argument was the unacceptable dilemma that might otherwise be created for the doctor if the parents could not consent to medical treatment when the child refused consent:[166]

> "If the position in law is that upon the achievement of 'Gillick competence' there is a transfer of the right of consent from parents to child and there can never be a concurrent right in both, doctors would be faced with an intolerable dilemma. On pain, if they got it wrong, of being sued for trespass to the person or possibly being charged with a criminal assault, they would have to determine as a matter of law in whom the right of consent resided at the particular time in relation to the particular treatment."

The "doctor's dilemma" is a familiar *cri de coeur* of the courts[167] but, arguably, it misrepresents the doctor's legal position. He is, in fact, in no greater dilemma than in many situations. First, after *Gillick* a doctor may act on the consent of a competent child patient and, therefore, he has to determine whether the child is competent to consent. While this may be no easy matter, it is no more difficult to determine a child's competence when the child is refusing treatment. Indeed, arguably the *Gillick* case creates a greater legal exposure were he to make a mistake in respect of a child's competence. If a doctor treated an incompetent child, it is far from clear that his reasonable mistake as to her competence would be a defence to a battery action.[168] If, however, a doctor were to wrongly determine that a child was competent and respected her refusal of treatment, his only liability could be in the tort of negligence for any resulting harm. Here, a reasonable mistake as to the child's competence would be a defence. In other words, it is the *Gillick* decision which creates the doctor's "intolerable dilemma". Accepting that a competent child may refuse treatment does not.

There are two final comments on this aspect of the case. First, if Lord Donaldson is correct, then a doctor *may* always look to a competent child's parents for confirmation (or rejection) of the child's decision. The effect of this would be, of course, to put the doctor in the position, or "dilemma" if you like, of choosing between the decision of the parents and the child if they are in disagreement. Whether the parents agree with the child's decision to consent or his refusal, Lord Donaldson does, in effect, give them a veto or, at least, a "trump card" in the decision-making process. Is this not giving them the power "to determine" – the very power which the House of Lords in *Gillick* denied them?[169]

Secondly, Lord Donaldson's approach raises significant problems in relation to confidentiality. How will parents be able to decide whether to exercise their power to consent? Clearly, they should be provided with the information which the doctor has in order to exercise this new-found power. However, the child will be, by definition, competent and, prima facie entitled to have his or her confidences respected. The doctor must break his confidence to inform the parents or he will deprive them of their opportunity ("right") to decide.

What is the doctor's position? He cannot have a duty to break the confidence because it is difficult, perhaps impossible, to frame the legal wrong to (and cause of action of) the parents. Remember, the Court of Appeal has recently held that there is no such thing as an action for infringement of parental rights.[170] Surely, there cannot be a legal duty which is unenforceable? So, at best the doctor has a discretion to inform the parents and break his child patient's confidence which can be done only if he views telling them as in the child's "best interests".[171]

The confidentiality point is a major issue not referred to in *re R*, which necessarily contemplates a sharing of information between the doctor and the child's parents. Arguably, the common law position (which must be assumed if Lord Donaldson is correct) will not march in step with Parliamentary intention. The Access to Health Records Act 1990 prevents a parent obtaining access to the child's medical records if the child is competent unless that child has consented to the parent gaining access (section 4(2)). Surely, therefore, the law should not allow a doctor to disclose voluntarily information in precisely these circumstances?

In conclusion then, if Lord Donaldson is correct, his view of parental power will run a "coach and horses" through the *Gillick* decision and the widely accepted view that the House of Lords was seeking to enfranchise children and recognise that in modern society competent children have the right to decide. If Lord Donaldson is correct, they only have the right to say "yes"!

The court and the competent child After the *Gillick* decision it was unclear whether a court in wardship (or exercising its inherent jurisdiction) could act against the wishes of a competent child and, for example, consent to medical treatment that the child refused.[172] One view of the court's wardship jurisdiction (and, perhaps, its wider inherent jurisdiction also) is that it steps into the shoes of the parents (or those with "parental responsibility") and the court then acts as a "prudent parent".[173] On this view, the powers of the court are those of the parents. Of course, there are a number of enforcement powers that are unique to the court (e.g. injunctions to prevent publication of any material that would identify a ward)[174] but these are not matters that go to the substance of the court's power. On this view, therefore, if the *Gillick* decision means that parents lose the power to consent to medical treatment when a child reaches a state of development when he or she is competent to consent, so does the court.

Another view of the court's jurisdiction is, however, possible. While the court acts as a judicial parent this is merely an analogy describing *how* it acts. The jurisdiction of the court is, however, not derived from the parents' powers over their child but is wider in scope, allowing the court to do anything that is necessary to protect the child. Consequently, a court may do what a parent cannot do if that is in the child's "best interests".[175] Thus, in a number of first instance cases, the court has taken account of a competent child's wishes in determining whether to authorise medical treatment but the court did not consider itself bound by the child's wishes if this conflicted with the court's view of the child's "best interests".[176]

In *re R* the Court of Appeal approved the second view of the court's jurisdiction and affirmed this line of first instance decisions. All three judges concluded that *Gillick* was not a wardship case and what was said by the House of Lords in that case was not intended to apply to the court's *parens patriae* jurisdiction. Lord Donaldson rejected the view that wardship derived from the parents' powers and responsibilities over their children and, therefore, was itself fettered by *Gillick*.[177] Instead, in his view, it arose from "the delegated performance of the duties of the Crown to protect its subjects and particularly children who are the generations of the future".[178] Hence, the court could act in the child's "best interests" if necessary by overriding the child's decision competently arrived at.[179] Staughton and Farquharson LJJ agreed.[180] Logically, on this view, the court would override the wishes of a competent adult if the court's *parens patriae* power of adults were to be restored in the future unless the court were specifically prohibiting from doing so by legislation!

On the whole, *re R* is consistent with the approach of the Children Act 1989.[181] By virtue of section 1(1) of the 1989 Act, the court in any proceedings concerning "the upbringing of a child" is required to consider "the child's welfare" as the "paramount consideration". Section 1(3) then goes on to provide a list of factors which a court shall have regard to in determining this issue, the first of which is stated in section 1(3)(a) to be "the ascertainable wishes and feelings of the child concerned (considered in the light of his age and understanding)". Clearly, therefore, a competent child's wishes are relevant but they do not appear to be conclusive.[182] This applies to wardship (including the wider inherent jurisdiction of the court). It also applies to a court making a "section 8 order",[183] a care order,[184] a child assessment order[185] and an emergency protection order.[186]

By contrast, in a number of instances under the 1989 Act a medical or psychiatric examination may be authorised by the court in the "best interests" of the child but it is recognised that a competent child has a right to refuse these medical interventions. So, for example, a court may not include a requirement in a "supervision order" made under section 31 that a child submit to a psychiatric or medical examination[187] or submit to psychiatric or medical treatment[188] when a child is competent to understand unless the child consents. Further, a child assessment order under section 43 may authorise a person to examine a child, but section 43(8) expressly states that "if the child is of sufficient understanding to make an informed decision he may refuse to submit to a medical or psychiatric examination or other assessment".[189]

In short, therefore, the 1989 Act consistently requires the competent child's views to be taken into account. While the general provisions of section 1(3) do not *require in every case* that the child's wishes be determinative, it does not, on the other hand, state that they cannot be. In a case where medical intervention is against the wishes of a child, surely the coercive nature of such intervention and the resulting insult to the dignity of the child ought to lead the court to not only have regard to the child's wishes, but also to make those wishes conclusive. This would, it is suggested, be quite consistent with section 1(3) of the 1989 Act.

What are the implications of *re R* when the court acts against the wishes of a competent child? There are two situations which might arise: (1) the court gives its consent when the child refuses treatment: (2) the court refuses to consent to (or even prohibits) treatment when the child consents.

In the first situation, the authority of the court would make any treatment (in the child's "best interests") lawful. It is another matter as to whether a doctor will carry out the treatment.[190] This will be a matter of his duty to treat, which turns upon his duty to exercise reasonable care and to act in the child's "best interests", taking account of the fact that the child is refusing treatment.[191] Further, it may be, in practical terms, impossible to give the treatment without the child's agreement.

The second situation is slightly different. If the court has refused its consent to (or prohibited the) treatment, then any action by a doctor will potentially be a contempt of court even if the child consents. Only Staughton LJ expressly dealt with this situation, but the logic of the approach in *re R* can lead nowhere else. If the child's "best interests" lead the court to consider treatment undesirable, then in exercising its protective jurisdiction the court should have the power to, in effect, ban treatment.

Conclusion

The family is the natural decision-maker for incompetent patients and it has been argued that this should be recognised in law not only in the case of children but also for adults. The family's role may have to give way to court review when doubt or disagreement exists, where the State's duty to protect those who are unable to protect themselves overrides the family's presumptive role and obligations. The court's role should, however, be seen in its proper context: first, through its legislative function in establishing society's criteria for valid decision-making and, secondly, by reviewing or supervising the decisions made on behalf of incompetent patients. It has been argued that this latter function should not be seen as an invitation to the court to descend into the decision-making arena such that the court becomes the decision-maker. What is true in the case of incompetent patients has to be the case for the competent. But, in *re R*, the Court of Appeal accepted the view that the court's *parens patriae* power exists not only to protect children from harm by others, but also to protect them from harm brought about by their own decisions. The Crown's power existed to prevent harm to individuals who are unable to care for themselves.[192] Arguably, the court's philosophy is out of step with the post-*Gillick* era, which turns its face against parental paternalism. It seems, however, that state paternalism is to be sanctioned and, while this is a philosophy which has received some, albeit, not whole-hearted support in the Children Act, it remains nonetheless difficult to support without specific Parliamentary approval.

Postscript

Since this paper was written, in *re W (a minor) (refusal of medical treatment)*[193] the Court of Appeal has considered again the scope of the court's powers and that of parents to consent to medical treatment in respect of teenage children who are competent to consent to medical treatment and who have refused their consent. The Court of Appeal reaffirmed its earlier decision in *re R*.

The Court held: (1) that a court had power, in certain circumstances, under its inherent power to override the refusal of a competent child; (2) that a parent (or other *in loco parentis*) could override the refusal of treatment by a competent child (per Lord Donaldson MR and Balcombe LJ; Nolan LJ dubitante).

The facts and background

W was a sixteen-year-old girl who suffered from anorexia nervosa, an eating disorder associated usually with the individual's desire to remain looking youthful, even child-like.[194] The individual will have a distorted perception of his or her body size and the condition manifests itself in an obsession with the individual's weight and the compulsion to lose weight, which is achieved through a refusal to eat food. The explanation for anorexia is unclear, but it is thought to be behavioural in origin, the individual resorting to a "relentless pursuit of excessive thinness"[195] in order to establish control over his or her life.[196] The condition itself is not fatal although, of course, starvation will ultimately result in death if the individual does not capitulate and eat. In addition, severe physical damage may result from the individual's self-imposed starvation, for example, there may be damage to the individual's reproductive organs, kidneys or even heart.[197]

W had a history of family tragedy and, because of the death of both her parents, was in local authority care. She had psychological problems over a long period and her anorexia nervosa first manifested itself in 1990. In 1991 she was admitted to a specialist residential unit for children and adolescents suffering from anorexia nervosa where she received treatment and at one time a nasogastric tube was used (with her consent) to feed her. Fearing that W might refuse further treatment, the local authority made an application to the High Court for the court to exercise its inherent jurisdication (wardship was, of course, unavailable because of section 100(2) (c) of the Children Act 1989) so as to permit the local authority to consent to such treatment as was necessary even if W refused that treatment.[198]

When the case came before Thorpe J the medical evidence did not disclose that W's life was threatened by her condition. Instead, the disagreement concerned where W was to be treated. She wished to remain in the residential unit where she currently lived (and there was support in the expert evidence for this continuing). However, another view of one consultant was that she should be moved to a specialist clinic in London for treatment including, if necessary, treatment against her wishes. Thorpe J found that "there is no doubt that W is a child of sufficient understanding to make an informed decision" but that following *re R*, the court was not bound by the wishes of a competent child.[199] Faced with the conflict of professional opinion, Thorpe J determined that it was in W's best interests to be treated at the specialist clinic and authorised her removal and treatment there regardless of her wishes.

By the time the case reached the Court of Appeal, W's condition had deteriorated considerably, such that the evidence indicated that "within a week her capacity to have children in later life would be seriously at risk and a little later her life might be in danger" (per Lord Donaldson MR).[200] Faced with this, the Court of Appeal issued an interim order authorising her removal to the specialist hospital and treatment. In effect, this determined the main issue in the appeal, that is, whether the court has power to authorise treatment under its inherent jurisdiction when a competent child refuses treatment. Nevertheless, the court continued to hear argument on the scope of this power (was it, for instance, to be restricted to situations where the child's life was threatened) and the related issue of the parental powers in cases where a competent child refuses treatment.

The court and the competent child

It is clear, as the interim order vouchsafed, that the court has the power under its inherent jurisdiction (including wardship) to consent to medical treatment when a "*Gillick*-competent" child refuses treatment. The court approved *re R* in this regard and reiterated the well known position, stated by Sir John Pennycuick in *re X (a minor)*,[201] that the court's powers are *theoretically* without limit. In the case of children who are 16 or over, the court rejected the argument that section 8 of the Family Law Reform Act 1969 pre-empted the court's inherent power.[202] This seems a weak argument and, in any event, as we shall see below, the judges held that section 8 did not even deal with the situation. It permitted a child age 16 or over to consent to medical treatment but did not give that child a right to refuse treatment.[203]

Nevertheless, this should not have led the court to view its powers as extending to cases like *re R* and *re W*. There are a number of principled reasons for this which go beyond a crude reliance on section 8.

First, as I suggested above, the court does not have (and never has had) a limitless power over competent children. The *parens patriae* power of the Crown extended to those who were unable to take care of themselves through their incompetence or physical incapacity. The prerogative jurisdiction over "lunatics, idiots, and others of unsound mind" was just what it says, a royal jurisdiction to take care of those members of society who needed care because they were *unable* to care for themselves, not because they were *unwilling* to do so.[204] Surely, wardship and the wider inherent jurisdiction (revitalised by the Children Act) as the direct descendants of this power must be of a similar scope? Any other view would lead to what I would suggest would be a wholly unacceptable position for any court to take, namely that the court may force medical care (or, indeed, anything) on any subject of the Crown simply because the court thinks that individual is in need of care. This should not be the law because it is unsound in theory and policy in a democratic society where notions of individual liberty are generally recognised and respected.

The Court of Appeal subsequently embodied just this policy in the law in the case of *re T (refusal of treatment)*[205] where a competent adult's legal right to refuse treatment, even where life is threatened, was emphatically stated by all the judges.[206] The social and public policy embodied in that decision sits uneasily with the view that the court may override the treatment decision of a competent child. Competent children are adults for these purposes. They are not *unable* to care for themselves, in these circumstances they are just *unwilling* to do so in a way that others think is best for them.

Secondly, as the judges themselves accepted in *re W*, the *theoretically* limitless powers of the court, if that is what they are, are *in practice* restricted by practical considerations,[207] by self-imposed fetters,[208] and by Parliamentary intervention.[209] Even if it is accepted that the power exists, the question in *re R* and *re W* was – *should the court limit its power*? The above arguments relying on notions of individual liberty and autonomy strongly (in my view conclusively) point in the direction of the court staying its hand. At best, this should be a question for Parliament. This latter point is important because the courts do not assume coercive powers of detention or treatment over competent members of society who are not a danger to others.[210] When the state wishes to act coercively against such a person, and this is fortunately a relatively infrequent occurrence, legislation is generally required. Hence, in the case of the mentally ill, the power to act is conferred by Parliament.[211] In this rare instance even individuals who are a danger *to themselves* may be dealt with against their wishes and their mental illness treated for their own good under the provisions in Part IV of the Mental Health Act 1983. Even though this is a wholly exceptional policy, W was, nevertheless, in effect treated by the Court of Appeal as if she were mentally ill and in need of treatment. Arguably, she was mentally ill and could have been treated under the Mental Health Act 1983, providing that the appropriate procedures were followed, even through Lord Donaldson, for some reason, doubted whether this was possible.[212] Then, of course, the statutory safeguards would have applied and the more general public policy in respect of the mentally ill would have been called into play. W may even have been incompetent to make a treatment decision. Only Lord Donaldson MR doubted Thorpe J's view that she understood and was, therefore, competent.[213] Lord Donaldson observed that one of the features of anorexia is that it is addictive and compulsive, such that the individual may have no control over the decision whether to eat or not. If this were the case, and it certainly looks plausible, then *re W* falls squarely within that category of case – the incompetent mentally ill patient – where it is accepted that coercive therapeutic intervention is justified. The case would have little legal value as a novel precedent seen in that light. But that was not the light, of course, in which the Court of Appeal viewed their decision.

A third reason why the court should not have authorised treatment against W's wishes stems from a proper perception of the function of the court in a wardship or inherent jurisdiction case. As I claimed above (see pp. 48–54), in proxy decision cases the role of the court should be twofold: initially, a legislative one (setting the criteria for making a treatment decision) and ultimately, a review one (ensuring that the correct criteria have been applied in a reasonable or rational manner). The court is in real difficulty in performing either of these functions when the treatment decision is not made by a proxy (a parent or doctor as a quasi-proxy) but by the patient herself. What are the criteria that a patient should use in making her own decision? Perhaps a patient should act in her own best interests. To this extent the court may act legislatively, but tells us (or the patient) little: certainly the patient is unlikely to need a court to tell her this. The court could, of course, specify that a patient must act in her best interests so as not to threaten her own life. A patient would thus be legislatively (through the court) mandated to act to choose life over death. But this, as we know from *re T*, the court will not do. A patient is left to her own death if that is her view of her best interests.[214] Further, were a court to attempt to perform its review function, its only option would be to ignore the patient's view of her own best interests and act on the basis of some overriding criterion – for example, the state interest in preserving life – but this would be to reach a conclusion expressly rejected in *re T*. It is quite legitimate for the court to set and police the application of society's criteria for proxy decision-making because it is acting to protect the vulnerable in the case of immature children or incompetent adults (see above, pp. 45–48). It is quite another matter to do so in the case of personal decision-making, whether by a competent child or adult. In this respect *re W* and *re T* cannot both stand; they are simply inconsistent.

The problems faced by a court in determining where a competent patient's best interests lie is illustrated by the way in which the judges in *re W* sought to take account of W's wishes. Although the judges all recognised that her wishes were not conclusive, it was also accepted that her wishes were relevant. Given that an "objective" observer (the court) would regard treatment as in the individual's best interests, how does the court "take account of" and "give due weight to" the wishes of the competent child who is refusing treatment? "With great difficulty" might be the short answer, since the court is really trying to compare two incompatibles—apples against oranges, if you like. She wants "X"; the court thinks "Y" is in her best interests. There is nothing here but for the court to accept that the factors leading to "Y" are simply more important than her wishes and so outweigh them. Surely this is a strange way to take account of her wishes if it will necessarily result (and it will) in them being overridden by, for example, the court's desire to save her from herself and keep her alive?

In *re W* Lord Donaldson MR stated that a child's wishes were relevant to an extent which was prudent but that:

> "Prudence does not involve avoiding all risk, but it does involve avoiding taking risks which, if they eventuate, may have irreparable consequences or which are disproportionate to the benefits which could accrue from taking them."

On the facts, he was content to state that, in reaching his decision, Thorpe J "was not only bearing W's wishes in mind, but looking behind them to see why W wished to remain where she was". Given that there was credible medical evidence which supported her choice and that her life was not then at risk, what are we to make of the weight Thorpe J gave to her wishes? It would appear that Lord Donaldson would contemplate a competent child's wishes being overriden in a wide range of situations where medical evidence (and the court) supported treatment.

By contrast, Balcombe LJ took a narrower view of the court's power to override a competent child's decision and, consequently, he gave the child's wishes much greater weight, perhaps even conclusive weight, in non-life-threatening situations. He created, in effect, a presumption in favour of the child's decision. Of course, in doing so he removes the need to "take account" of the child's wishes and balance them against competing interests. He stated:

> "It will normally be in the best interests of a child of sufficient understanding to make an informed decision that the court should respect its integrity as a human being and not lightly override its decision on such a personal matter as medical treatment, all the more so if that treatment is invasive. In my judgment, therefore, the court exercising the inherent jurisdiction in relation to a 16 or 17-year-old child who is not mentally incompetent will, as a matter of course, ascertain the wishes of the child and will approach its decision with a strong predilection to give effect to the child's wishes ... Nevertheless, if the court's powers are to be meaningful, there must come a point at which the court, while not disregarding the child's wishes, can override them in the child's best interests, objectively considered. Clearly such a point will have come if the child is seeking to refuse treatment in circumstances which will in all probability lead to the death of the child or to severe permanent injury."

On this basis, Balcombe LJ (alone) thought that Thorpe J had reached the wrong decision in overriding W's wishes, since he had given them insufficient weight at a time when her life was not threatened. Of course, the Court of Appeal was faced with a situation where W's life was at risk.

Given the difference between the wider view of Lord Donaldson and the narrower view of Balcombe LJ, what of the third judge, Nolan LJ? His position is curious for its internal inconsistency. Nolan LJ expressly rejected the argument of the Official Solicitor which would have restricted the court's powers to override a competent child's wishes to, *inter alia*, those situations where the procedure was "necessary to prolong or save the child's life or to protect the child from really serious and irreparable harm". On the face of it, therefore, one would expect his view to be close to the wider power espoused by Lord Donaldson. The remainder of his judgment is, on the contrary, close to the narrower view of Balcombe LJ. In words reminiscent of Balcombe LJ, Nolan LJ stated:

> "I am very far from asserting any general rule that the court should prefer its own view as to what is in the best interests of the child to those of the child itself. In considering the welfare of the child, the court must not only recognise but if necessary defend the right of the child, having sufficient understanding to take an informed decision, to make his or her own choice. In most areas of life it would not only be wrong in principle but also futile and counter-productive for the Court to adopt any different approach."

Like Balcombe LJ, Nolan LJ saw the court as entitled to act for the "protection of the child's life" because "it is the duty of the Court to ensure so far as it can that children survive to attain [the age of 18]". Consequently, the court has a duty to intervene where there is "a serious and imminent risk that the child will suffer grave and irreversible mental or physical harm ... Due weight must be given to the child's wishes, but the Court is not bound by them". On the facts, however, Nolan LJ supported Thorpe J's initial decision, but only the premise that such a risk existed (which is doubtful).

Will the difference in emphasis of the judges affect the outcome of a case? It is unlikely given the scope of the Balcombe LJ/Nolan LJ category covering cases where life or limb is threatened. Rarely will cases come before the courts where the child's life or limb is not at stake. These are the controversial cases where doctors, parents and others concerned about the child's welfare instinctively feel the child is making the wrong decision and hence seek the court's assistance. In these cases, the state interest in preserving life seems, according to *re W*, to trump the individual interests of the competent child (although not of the competent adult). The result is that *re W* has enshrined state paternalism until such time that the House of Lords is called upon to review *re R* and *re W*.

Parents and the competent child

One of the most controversial aspects of *re R* was, as we saw, the dictum by Lord Donaldson that a parent had power to authorise medical treatment in the face of a refusal by a competent child. Although strictly not necessary for the decision in *re W*, both Lord Donaldson MR (perhaps not surprisingly) and also Balcombe LJ affirmed the Master of the Rolls' dictum in *re R*. I have set out the arguments against this position at some length above (pp. 59–65) and nothing would be gained by repeating them here. However, some comments are in order.

Unlike R, it will be recalled that W was 16 years of age. Hence, in *re W* the court was required to consider in detail the effect of section 8 of the Family Law Reform Act 1969.[215] In doing so, Lord Donaldson and Balcombe LJ interpreted it narrowly. For them, section 8 was enacted in order to protect a doctor from civil and criminal liability for assault or battery if he treated a child aged between 16 and 18 without parental consent. It acted, in the words of Lord Donaldson, as a "flak jacket" for the medical profession. Further, section 8 spoke only of the child's *right to consent*, it said nothing about refusal and was not intended to.[216] In other words, section 8 did not affect the legal position of the parents, who retain a continuing "right" to consent to treatment on a child up to the age of 18.

Rarely can a court have so effectively emasculated a position which has come to gain almost unanimous support outside the courts.[217] The "settled interpretation" of section 8 (as it was referred to by Balcombe LJ) – more accurately perhaps put as the "accepted interpretation" – was treated with nothing short of contempt by the judges because it had never been stated by a judge but only by legal commentators.[218] One can only guess whether a casual comment of the Benchers over lunch in the Inns would carry more weight than the considered view of the academicians! Of course, the House of Lords did consider the meaning of section 8 in *Gillick*, as I pointed out above. The judges in *re W* dismissed the Law Lords' views as *obiter dicta*, section 8 being irrevelant in *Gillick*. Again, in *re W* the judges emphasised section 8(3), which for them reserved the parents' power to consent, notwithstanding the child's right conferred by section 8(1). Section 8(3), it will be recalled, states that:

> "Nothing in this section shall be construed as making ineffective any consent which would have been effective if this section had not been enacted."

This provision, of course, allowed the House of Lords in *Gillick* to give effect to the common law notion of competence to consent for children who are *under 16* and who, therefore, are not covered by section 8. Section 8(3) is, at best, ambiguous as to whether it preserves the right of another to consent in the case of a *post-16*-year-old child, i.e. consent by the parents. It is the effect of *Gillick* which gives guidance on whether a parent may consent to treatment once the child is competent and thus, what is left to be recognised by section 8(3).

Finally in *re W*, the House of Lords' decision in *Gillick* was, as in *re R*, restricted to empowering a competent child (of any age) to consent while not affecting a parent's concurrent right to consent in the face of a refusal by the child. While not treated with contempt, *Gillick* was subjected to the kind of nit-picking scrutiny (analysis would be too grand) reminiscent of that once adopted in relation to tax statutes by the House of Lords. Only Lord Scarman's speech could be interpreted as having contemplated the *re R* and *re W* situation and, even if he did, which he probably did not (per Lord Donaldson MR and Balcombe LJ), no-one else in *Gillick* contemplated it.[219] On this basis, *Gillick* was only concerned with, to repeat the words of Lord Donaldson, providing a "flak jacket" to the doctor. *Gillick* was, therefore, according to Lord Donaldson MR and Balcombe LJ, simply irrelevant.

On this type of analysis most of *re R* and *re W* would not survive as authority for anything important concerning the interrelationship between parents and their children which was not strictly at issue. Nolan LJ had the good sense and wisdom to distance himself from the views of the other judges. For him, cases of disagreement between children who are competent and their parents over medical treatment could only be resolved by the court. Of course, we know what the court would do with the child's wishes in such a case! At least, it would only be state, rather than parental, paternalism.

The legal position espoused by Lord Donaldson and Balcombe LJ creates the spectre of children undergoing invasive medical procedures against their wishes but with their parents' consent. Imagine the situation, raised in *re W*, of the pregnant girl aged under 16 but "*Gillick*-competent", or aged between 16 and 18, who wishes to keep her child but whose parents believe this would not be in her best interests. Legally a doctor could act on the consent of the parents alone. Is it sufficient for Lord Donaldson and Balcombe LJ to state that:

> "I cannot conceive of a case where a doctor ... would terminate the pregnancy merely upon the consent of the girl's parents" (per Balcombe LJ).

Surely we are here in the realm of fundamental rights? I do not mean the right to procreate or have a family but the far more basic right to be "left alone". Courts should protect such rights of competent individuals whether child or adult. *Re T* seeks to give effect to such a right and both Balcombe and Nolan LJJ acknowledged its importance for the court. Surely, it is essential to do so between parent and child also?

Re W should be overruled by the House of Lords in all its respects but in particular in its suborning of a child's rights to the (otherwise) discredited "rights" of parents. *Re W*, like Lord

Donaldson in *re R* before, places decision-making power in the wrong hands.

Notes and references

1. *Schloendorff* v. *Society of New York Hospital* (1914) 105 NE 92 at 93. Cardozo CJ (by then Chief Justice of the New York Court of Appeals) was appointed to the United States Supreme Court in 1932, succeeding Oliver Wendell Holmes. For a discussion of the appointments and tenure of these two jurists, see H. Abraham, *Justices & Presidents* (1985) chs 8 and 9, and for a discussion of Cardozo's contribution as a torts' jurist see G. Edward White, *Tort Law in America* (1980) ch. 4).
2. [1985] 1 All ER 643 at 649. See also Lord Bridge at 660; and per Lord Templeman at 66.
3. Ibid.
4. [1990] 2 AC 1 at 12 per Lord Donaldson MR. See also, at 29–30 per Neill LJ, at 35–6 per Butler-Sloss LJ, at 55 per Lord Brandon, at 72–3 per Lord Goff.
5. The extent to which a competent adult patient's refusal to consent to treatment may be overridden is controversial. See the discussion of the American case law in I. Kennedy and A. Grubb, *Medical Law: Text and Materials* (1989, Butterworth) at 346–64. The issue has not arisen in a modern English case although in *Re F (in utero)* [1988] 2 All ER 193 there is a strong hint by the Court of Appeal that the courts will require Parliament to sanction such coercive measures, as has occurred in the case of the mentally ill in the Mental Health Act 1983. See especially, Balcombe LJ at 200–3. Discussed, Grubb [1988] All ER Rev 200 at 212–13. See also I. Kennedy, *Treat Me Right* (1991, Oxford University Press) ch. 19.
6. For a fascinating discussion of the ethical basis of surrogate or proxy decision-making, see A. Buchanan and D. Brock *Deciding for Others: The Ethics of Surrogate Decision-Making* (1989). For a discussion of the legal principles, see I. Kennedy and A. Grubb, op cit at 290–345 (general principles) and 1086–1155 (dying patients).
7. See also King, "The authority of families to make medical decisions for incompetent patients after the Cruzan decision" (1991) 19 *Law, Medicine & Health Care* 76.
8. This would (and should) cover heterosexual couples who are not married and homosexual couples. As to the former note the approach of the Court of Appeal in *Dyson Holdings Ltd* v. *Fox* [1976] QB 503 and *Watson* v. *Lucas* [1980] 1 WLR 1493 (applying the inheritancy provisions of the protected tenancy legislation). As to the latter, see infra note 47.
9. See Mental Health Act 1983, s. 26 (defining "relative" and "nearest relative"). Notice also the definition of "member of another's

family" in s. 113(1) of the Housing Act 1985 – spouse, person living together as husband and wife, parent, grandparent, child, grandchild, brother, sister, uncle, aunt, nephew and niece.

10. Consultation Paper No. 119 (1991) at paras 6.1–6.61.
11. Ibid at paras 5.1–5.29. Others would include "durable powers of attorney" whereby the patient could formally appoint another to act on his behalf when the patient becomes incompetent. Although England has the Enduring Powers of Attorney Act 1985, this almost certainly does not cover health care decisions; see *The Living Will: Consent to Treatment at the End of Life* (1988, Edward Arnold) at 48–9 (Working Party Report of Centre of Medical Law and Ethics, King's College and Age Concern).
12. Meyers, "The family and life and death decisions" in *Family Rights: Family Law & Medical Advance* (eds E. Sutherland and A. McCall Smith) (1990, Edinburgh University Press) 59 at 63.
13. *In Re Quinlan* (1976) 355 A2d 647 (NJ Sup Ct).
14. See Susan Jinnett-Sack, "Autonomy in the company of others", this volume.
15. *Cruzan* v. *Director, Missouri Department of Health* (1990) 110 S Ct 2841 and (1990) 58 LW 4916 (US Sup Ct) (citation hereafter to the *Law Week* reference). For a discussion see Bryan Jennett and Susan Jinnett-Sack in this volume.
16. However, in many areas the "private realm of family life which the state cannot enter" without a compelling State interest is well recognised (*Prince* v. *Massachusetts* (1944) 321 US 158 at 166 per Rutledge J); see L. Tribe, *American Constitutional Law* (2nd edn, 1988) at 1414–20.
17. The exceptions are the States of Missouri (*Cruzan* v. *Harmon* (1988) 760 SW 2d 408 (Mo. Sup. Ct)) and New York (*In re Westchester County Medical Center (O'Connor)* (1988) 531 NE 2d 607 (NY CA)). Both refuse to allow the family of an incompetent adult patient to decide whether to withdraw life-sustaining treatment unless there is "clear and convincing evidence" that this was the patient's expressed wish prior to his becoming incompetent. It was this requirement that subsequently divided the US Supreme Court 5 votes to 4 in *Cruzan*, op cit The requirement has been welcomed by some (e.g. Bopp and Marzan, "Cruzan: facing the inevitable" (1991) 19 *Law, Medicine & Health Care* 37) but strongly rejected by others (e.g. Annas, "The long dying of Nancy Cruzan" (1991) 19 *Law, Medicine & Health Care* 52).
18. For a chart of the relevant State laws see Areen, "Advance directives under State law and judicial decisions" (1991) 19 *Law, Medicine & Health Care* 91 at 93–7.
19. President's Commission for the Study of Ethical Problems in Medicine and Biomedicine and Behavioural Research, *Deciding to Forego Life-Sustaining Treatment* (1983) passim, especially 127.
20. The proposition is best illustrated by the trilogy of New Jersey

Supreme Court decisions concerned with discontinuing life-sustaining treatment: *In re Conroy* (1985) 486 A2d 1209; *In re Peter* (1987) 539 A2d 419 and *In re Jobes* (1987) 529 A2d 434. In a fourth decision – *In re Farrell* (1987) 529 A2d 335 – the New Jersey Supreme Court held that a *competent* patient could decline life-sustaining treatment. For a discussion of these cases by a Justice of the New Jersey Supreme Court, see Pollock, "Life and death decisions: who makes them and by what standards" (1989) 41 *Rutgers Law Review* 505. The academic literature is voluminous, but for a comprehensive account, arguing for family decision-making, see Rhoden, "Litigating life and death" (1988) 102 *Harvard Law Review* 375 (for a contrary view see Dresser, "Relitigating life and death" (1990) 51 *Ohio State Law Journal* 425.

21. See Robertson, "Organ donation by incompetents and the substituted judgment doctrine" (1976) 76 *Columbia Law Review* 48. The historical basis is discussed by Robertson, op cit at 57–9. The application of "substituted judgment" is not without its detractors. See Dresser, "Life, death, and incompetent patients: conceptual infirmities and hidden values in the law" (1986) 28 *Arizona Law Review* 373 and Dresser and Robertson, "Quality of life and non-treatment decisions for incompetent patients: a critique of the orthodox approach" (1989) 17 *Law, Medicine & Health Care* 234.
22. (1989) 549 NE 2d 292 at 299 (permitting a guardian to refuse artificial hydration and nutrition for a seriously ill and incompetent patient applying a "substituted judgment" test). See also *in re Estate of Greenspan* (1990) 558 NE 2d 1194 (Ill Sup Ct) (applying *Longeway* and permitting a guardian to refuse artificial hydration and nutrition for a patient in a persistent vegetative state applying a "substituted judgment" test).
23. In *Brophy* v. *New England Sinai Hospital Inc.* (1986) 497 NE 2d 626 (Mass Sup Jud Ct) the following were taken into account in concluding that the incompetent patient would have wanted his food and hydration withdrawn: (1) expressed preferences; (2) religious convictions; (3) impact on his family; (4) probability of adverse side effects; (5) prognosis both with and without treatment; (6) the patient's present and future incompetence. For the development and use of "value histories" see Lambert, Gibson and Nathanson, "The values history: an innovation in surrogate medical decision-making" (1990) 18 *Law, Medicine & Health Care* 202.
24. *In re Storar* (1981) 420 NE 2d 64 (NY CA) (profoundly retarded patient of 52 with a mental age of 18 months since birth: "it is unrealistic to attempt to determine whether he would want to continue potentially life prolonging treatment if he were competent"). Cf. *Superintendent of Belchertown State School* v. *Saikewicz* (1977) 370 NE 2d 417 (Mass Sup Jud Ct) (67-year-old profoundly

retarded adult with a mental age of 2 years and eight months: court applied "substituted judgment" test).

25. See *Curran* v. *Bosze* (1990) 566 NE 2d 1319 (Ill Sup Ct) (substituted judgment test held inapplicable when court refused to order bone-marrow test on $3\frac{1}{2}$-year-old twins with a view to donation to their half-brother). This and other cases are discussed in Hunter, "Consent for the legally incompetent organ donor" (1991) 12 *Journal of Legal Medicine* 535. Contrast *re J (a minor) (wardship: medical treatment)* [1990] 3 All ER 930 (applying "substituted judgment" to a newborn baby) and for criticism see Grubb [1990] All ER Rev 182 at 185–7.
26. See President's Commission, supra note 19 at 132–4.
27. See Areen, op cit
28. Decisions of a properly appointed proxy/surrogate decision-maker may be constitutionally protected: see *Cruzan*, op cit at 4924 (O'Connor J concurring).
29. E.g. South Carolina: SC Code 1990 sections 44-66-10 to 80.
30. The position in Scotland is different because the court may appoint a tutor-dative to act on behalf of an incompetent adult: see *Dick* v. *Douglas* 1924 SLT 578 and Ward, "Revival of tutor-dative" 1987 SLT (News) 69.
31. For a very thought-provoking discussion see B. Hoggett and D. Pearl, *The Family, Law and Society: Cases and Materials* (3rd edn 1991, Butterworth) ch. 1.
32. [1990] 2 AC 1 (HL).
33. For a discussion see I. Kennedy, *Treat Me Right* (1991 paperback) ch. 20 and Grubb [1989] All ER Rev 200–6.
34. See especially Lord Goff's speech, ibid at 74–8.
35. This is the received wisdom: see Grubb and Pearl, "Sterilisation and the courts" [1987] CLJ 439 at 456–7. See also, P. D. G. Skegg, *Law, Medicine and Ethics* (1984) at 72–3. Cf. *Wilson* v. *Pringle* [1986] 2 All ER 440 at 447 per Croom-Johnson LJ (wrongly assuming next of kin could provide a valid consent).
36. B. Furrow, S. Johnson, T. Jost and R. Schwartz, *Health Law: Cases, Materials and Problems* (1991, 2nd edn, West) at 1129. See *Canterbury* v. *Spence* (1972) 464 F2d 772 at 789 per Robinson J.
37. *Gillick* v. *West Norfolk and Wisbech AHA* [1985] 3 All ER 402, especially per Lord Scarman at 419–21.
38. Ibid at 421 per Lord Scarman.
39. Notice cases such as *R* v. *Stone and Dobinson* [1977] QB 354 and *R* v. *Smith* [1979] Crim LR 251 (manslaughter charges based upon a legal duty of the "carer" owed to the infirmed or incompetent patient).
40. Ibid at 78 per Lord Goff.
41. Ibid per Lord Goff at 78. See also per Lord Bridge at 52; per Lord Brandon at 68; per Lord Griffiths at 69; per Lord Jauncey at 83–4.

42. Supra per Lord Brandon at 55–6; per Lord Goff at 77 (but cf. 77–8). In *re T (refusal of treatment)* (1992) 30 July (CA), Lord Donaldson MR appeared to reject both the notion of family decision-makers and, as regards the doctors, the test of "substituted judgement".
43. *Ex parte Whitbread, a Lunatic* (1816) 2 Mer Rep 99.
44. [1991] 3 All ER 866 (Hoffman J).
45. See also *re D(J)* [1982] 2 All ER 37 at 42–3. Megarry V-C stated that in making a will or authorising as an *inter vivos* gift under (what are now) sections 96(1)(c) and (d) of the Mental Health Act 1983, the court should approach the issue on the following basis:
(1) it is to be assumed that the patient is having a brief lucid interval;
(2) the patient, at that time, is to be assumed to have full knowledge of the fact that he will relapse into the mental state that actually exists;
(3) the court is to consider the position of the *actual* patient including any idiosyncrasies he might have had;
(4) during the hypothetical lucid period the patient is to be assumed to be receiving legal advice.
See generally, Heywood and Massey, *Court of Protection Practice*, (ed. N. Whitehorn) (12th edn 1991) at 191–201.
46. A. Buchanan and D. Brock, op cit at 136.
47. But contrast *re Wirdesedt* [1990] Imm AR 20 (CA) (homosexual partner not a "close relative"); *Harrogate BC* v. *Simpson* [1986] 2 FLR 91 (CA) (homosexual (female) partner not a "member of the tenant's family" under s. 113 of the Housing Act 1985).
48. See *in re Nemser* (1966) 273 NYS 2d 624 (NY Sup Ct) (disagreement between two sons over whether the leg of 80-year-old mother should be amputated).
49. See President's Commission Report, op cit at 128–9.
50. The dissenting justices took issue with the majority's view that abuse or erroneous decision-making warranted a "clear and convincing" evidential standard. For Brennan J maintaining the status quo of a patient (if erroneous) would degrade his existence and perpetuate the family's suffering. The rejection of "other" evidence of the patient's wishes evinced distain for the patient's right to choose (*supra* at 4931). Further, by allowing the State to require such a high level of proof on the basis of the State's interest in "preserving life", the majority was not safeguarding the patient's choice but "simply appropriating it" (supra at 4933).
51. Supra at 4920–1.
52. Supra at 4922.
53. Supra at 4921 per Rehnquist CJ.
54. See e.g. Brennan J (dissenting) in *Cruzan* supra at 4932: "Family members have a unique knowledge of the patient which is vital to any decision on his or her behalf."

55. *In re Quinlan* (1976) 355 A2d 647 (NJ Sup Ct).
56. E.g. *In re Guardianship of Hamlin* (1984) 689 P2d 1372 (Wash Sup Ct). But note *in re Guardianship of Grant* (1987) 747 P2d 445 (Wash Sup Ct); corrected (1988) 757 P2d 534. In *in re Conroy* (1985) 486 A2d 1209 the New Jersey Supreme Court required the involvement of the State nursing home ombudsman where the patient is in a nursing home.
57. See McCall Smith, "Committee ethics? Clinical ethics committees and their introduction in the United Kingdom" (1990) 17 *Journal of Law and Society* 124.
58. See Claire Gilbert Foster's chapter in this volume.
59. See infra, text to notes 76–82.
60. Supra, per Lord Brandon at 57–8; per Lord Griffiths at 70; per Lord Goff at 71. It remains unclear whether the Mental Health Act 1959 impliedly repealed (strictly put into abeyance) the Crown's prerogative or whether the revocation of the Royal Warrant delegating the power to the judges simply devested the judges. The judges in *re F* do not make the position clear. For a discussion see Hoggett, "The royal prerogative in relation to the mentally disordered: resurrection, resuscitation or rejection" in MDA Freeman (ed), *Medicine, Ethics and Law* (1988) at 85. See also Grubb and Pearl, op cit at 458–64.
61. *T* v. *T* [1988] 1 All ER 613 per Wood J at 625.
62. See Law Commission Consultation Paper No. 119 (1991), *Mentally Incapacitated Adults and Decision-Making: An Overview* at paras 3.35–3.36. There are procedural difficulties which would require legislation if the prerogative power could be (and was) restored by the Queen reissuing a Royal Warrant under the Sign Manual since the legislation regulating, for example, the procedure has been repealed. See Law Commission, ibid, and Grubb and Pearl, op cit at 462–4.
63. Op cit at 159.
64. For example, *re E (a minor)* (unreported, 21 September 1990, Ward J) (blood transfusion authorised against wishes of 15-year-old Jehovah's Witness). This case only came to light because it was cited in the subsequent Court of Appeal decision of *re R (a minor)* [1991] 4 All ER 177.
65. For example, *re F (a mental patient: sterilisation)* [1990] 2 AC 1 (only dispute concerned the jurisdiction of the court and the legal source of the doctor's power to sterilise a mentally handicapped adult woman. It was accepted by everyone that the procedure was in her "best interests": per Lord Brandon, supra at 54).
66. Supra at 140–1.
67. Supra at 160.
68. Supra at 141 *et seq.*
69. 1 *Blackstone's Commentaries* (17th edn 1830) vol 1, chs 16 and 17.

70. Vested in the mother and father jointly if married (s. 2(1)); and the mother alone if she is unmarried (s. 2(2)) unless imposed by the court on another (s. 4(1)).
71. It is important to notice the effect of the Children Act 1989. Where a court has made an interim or full care order under sections 31 or 38 of the Children Act 1989, parental responsibility vests in the local authority (s. 33(3)(a) – care order and, as a result of s. 31(11), this applies to interim care orders). A care order does not divest the parents of their "parental responsibility" for the child. Consequently, both they, and the local authority (who acquire parental responsibility as well under the order), concurrently have the power to make decisions (ss. 2(5) and (6)). However, the local authority may restrict the parents' "parental responsibility", including their ability to consent to (or refuse) medical treatment (s. 33(3)(b)).
72. See generally, Dickens, "The modern function and limits of parental rights" (1981) 97 LQR 462. Notice also that s. 3(5) of the Children Act 1989 would permit a person in whose care the child is (but who does not have parental responsibility) to consent to medical treatment that is "reasonable in the circumstances", for example, where the child was involved in an accident and consultation with the parents was impossible or impractical. Medical treatment that is not necessary for the child's welfare, in the sense that it is reasonable to seek the consent of those with "parental responsibility", would not fall within s. 3(5). See Law Commission, *Report on Guardianship and Custody* (No. 172, 1988) at para. 2.16.
73. [1985] 3 All ER 402. See I. Kennedy, *Treat Me Right* (1991; paperback edition) ch. 5.
74. See the discussion in *Department of Health & Community Services (NT)* v. *JWB and SMB* (1992) 66 ALJR 300 (Aust High Ct) especially at 338–40 per McHugh J.
75. *Re J (a minor) (wardship: medical treatment)* [1990] 3 All ER 930 at 934 per Lord Donaldson MR.
76. See, for example, the material collected in B. Hoggett and D. Pearl, op cit at 424–37.
77. The Children Act 1989 restricts the use of wardship. The following should be noted:

    (1) As a result of section 100(2)(c), wardship is not available in the case of a child who is in local authority care (s. 100(2)(b)). However, section 100 distinguishes between the court's inherent jurisdiction as *parens patriae* and the specific procedure of wardship under section 41 of the Supreme Court Act 1981 (and RSC Ord 90).

    (2) A local authority may, with the leave of the court, invoke the court's inherent jurisdiction to determine a specific question about a child's medical treatment.

    (3) Before granting leave, the court must be satisfied that there is

no other statutory order available, which there would not be, and that "there is reasonable cause to believe that if the court's inherent jurisdiction is not exercised ... the child ... is likely to suffer significant harm" (s. 100(3), (4) and (5)).

(4) Section 100(2)(d) prevents the court exercising its jurisdiction "for the purpose of conferring on any local authority power to determine any question ... in connection with any aspect of parental responsibility for a child". However, this does not seem to apply since the court is not conferring "power" on the local authority but merely determining what would be a proper course for the local authority subsequently to take in exercising its "parental responsibility" in respect of medical care of the child.

(5) If a child is not in the local authority's care, the local authority may not invoke the inherent jurisdiction of the court because the local authority would require the leave of the court under s. 100(3). But in such a case the requirement that the local authority could not achieve the same result through another statutory order would not be satisfied because, of course, a local authority may seek a "section 8 order" (with leave) or a care order under section 31 (or interim order under s. 38).

(6) The Act does not affect what is sometimes called "private wardship" cases. Hence the wardship (or wider inherent) jurisdiction of the court is available to a parent or health authority (which is not a "local authority" under the Act: s. 105(1)), if the child is not in care and may be invoked without the need to obtain the leave of the court.

(7) Alternatively, if the child is in care, the court's inherent jurisdiction can be invoked by a parent or health authority, again without leave, subject to the familiar and stringent limitations imposed by the House of Lords in *A* v. *Liverpool CC* [1982] AC 363 and *re W (a minor) (wardship: jurisdiction)* [1985] AC 791 before the Act when attempts were made to ward children in care. Of course, "section 8 orders" will also be available if the child is not in care but wardship (or the inherent jurisdiction) may be more advantageous in terms of speed and would be essential if the procedure is not a matter falling within "parental responsibility".

(8) The existence of a jurisdiction wider than wardship is controversial. There does not appear to be any procedure for invoking the court's inherent jurisdiction. But notice the suggestion in R. White, P. Carr and N. Lowe, *A Guide to the Children Act* (1990) at para. 10.5 that an application could be made by originating summons and headed "In the matter of the inherent jurisdiction". Wardship is usually taken as the *exclusive* procedure for invoking it (see, for example, *re F supra*, per Lord Griffiths at 70 and *re C (a minor) (wardship: medical treatment) (No. 2)* [1989] 2 All ER 791 at 793 per Lord Donaldson MR). By contrast, the Government

accepted the existence of a wider inherent jurisdiction and intended, after the Act, that it would be available to deal with difficult issues such as arise in the medical cases. See, for example, *In re J (a minor)* (1992) *The Times*, 15 May (Thorpe J).

(9) If there are medical procedures which parents cannot consent to, for example, sterilisation (see *re B (a minor) (wardship: sterilisation)* [1988] AC 199 at 205 per Lord Templeman), then the inherent jurisdiction is the only mechanism by which consent to such procedures can be obtained. It does not fall within the power or "parental responsibility" of parents or local authorities. As a consequence, they may not decide and, further, it does not fall within the "section 8 order" regime which is limited to matters relating to "parental responsibility" (s. 8(1)).

78. See, in general, *re S (infants)* [1967] 1 WLR 396 at 407 per Cross J. In the medical context see, for example, *re D (a minor) (wardship: sterilisation)* [1976] Fam 185 (sterilisation); *re P (a minor)* (1981) 80 LGR 301 (abortion and IUD). It is unclear whether this is true of the wider "inherent jurisdiction". It may be that here, unlike in wardship, the court only concerns itself with the "step" in the child's life referred to the court. Cf. *in re J (a minor)* (1992) *The Times* 15 May; Thorpe J considered that the power of the court exercising its inherent jurisdiction was "coextensive" with the power traditionally exercised in wardship.

79 A "section 8" order may be made in the course of any "family proceedings" (widely defined in ss. 8(3) and (4)) or, in a self-contained application, by some as of right (e.g. parents) or by others with the leave of the court having regard to their connection with the child (s. 10); the latter might include a doctor, social worker or health authority concerned about the child's medical care.

80. This would prevent a parent taking a particular (named) action without the consent of the court, for example, consenting to the disconnection of a life-support machine (see s. 8(1)).

81. Neither order can be made if the child is in the care of a local authority (s. 9(1)).

82. This has long been the judicial approach; see, for example, *re B (a minor) (wardship: sterilisation)* [1988] AC 199 (HL) and it is now reflected in section 1 of the Children Act 1989.

83. E.g. *Superintendent of Belchertown State School* v. *Saikewicz* (1977) 370 NE 2d 417 (Mass Sup Jud Ct); and *Eichner* v. *Dillon* (1980) 42 NYS 2d 517 (NY Sup Ct App Div). See Barron, "Medical paternalism and the rule of law: a reply to Dr Relman" (1979) 4 *American Journal of Law and Medicine* 337.

84. See *in re Spring* (1980) 405 NE 2d 115; *in re Dinnerstein* (1978) 380 NE 2d 134 (Mass App Ct); *re John Storar* (1981) 420 NE 2d 64 (NY CA); *Satz* v. *Perlmutter* (1980) 379 So2d 359 (Fla Sup Ct) and

Cruzan v. *Director, Missouri Department of Health* (1990) 110 S Ct 2841 at 2884 n.13 per Stevens J (dissenting). See the discussion in I. Kennedy and A. Grubb *Medical Law: Text and Materials* (1989) at 963–7.

85. [1988] AC 199. Discussed in Grubb and Pearl, op cit.
86. Ibid at 205–6. None of the other judges expressed a view on the requirement of court involvement.
87. See Grubb and Pearl, op cit at 452–6.
88. See supra, especially per Lord Goff at 79–80. See also per Lord Brandon at 56–7. Only Lord Griffiths adopted Lord Templeman's approach, supra at 70–1.
89. Supra at 56. He also referred to: (1) the irreversible nature of the operation; (2) the fact that it would deprive the woman of the fundamental right to bear children; (3) the moral and emotional considerations raised by sterilisation.
90. See, for example, *re B (a minor) (wardship: medical treatment)* (1981) [1990] 3 All ER 927 where the Court of Appeal authorised life-saving surgery on a newly born baby with Down's syndrome. Templeman LJ (at 928) emphasised the difficulty of the parents deciding when faced with the shock of giving birth to such a child. But cf. Dunn LJ (at 929) stating that their decision was "an entirely responsible one".
91. *F* v. *F* (1992) 7 BMLR 135 (Stephen Brown P) (29-year-old mentally handicapped woman undergoing hysterectomy for serious menorrhagia); *re E (a minor) (medical treatment)* (1992) 7 BMLR 117 (Stephen Brown P) (17-year-old mentally handicapped girl undergoing hysterectomy for same reasons). See also *re SG (a patient)* (1992) 6 BMLR 95 (Stephen Brown P) (No need to come to court when an abortion is proposed upon a 26-year-old mentally handicapped woman; the Abortion Act 1967 provided sufficient safeguards). Other "mandatory court cases" might involve such procedures as live organ donation or non-therapeutic research (see *re F* supra, per Neill LJ at 33; per Lord Bridge at 52). The former would, of course, have to be between "genetically related" individuals as defined in section 2(2) of the Human Organ Transplants Act 1989 since live organ donation by an incompetent person is otherwise prohibited by the Human Organ Transplants (Unrelated Persons) Regulations 1989 (SI No. 2480), Reg 3.
92. Contrast the position in Australia, where court approval is necessary for sterilisations of mentally handicapped girls or women because of their particular vulnerability and the danger of unintentional or intentional abuse by others: *Department of Health & Community Services (NT)* v. *JWB and SMB* (1992) 66 ALJR 300 (Aust High Ct) (Brennan, Deane and McHugh JJ dissenting).
93. See Dickens, op cit.

94. Discussed by Grubb [1989] All ER Rev 200 at 205–10 and [1990] All ER Rev 182 at 182–8.
95. [1990] 3 All ER 927.
96. [1989] 2 All ER 782.
97. [1990] 3 All ER 930.
98. Ibid at 934 (emphasis in original).
99. [1990] (1981) 3 All ER 927 at 929 per Templeman LJ.
100. [1976] Fam 185.
101. [1991] 2 FLR 426
102. See also, *re P (a minor)* (1981) 80 LGR 301 (consent to abortion on 15-year-old girl against parents' wishes).
103. McCall Smith, "Is anything left of parental rights?" in *Family Rights: Family Law and Medical Advance* (eds E. Sutherland and A. McCall Smith, 1990, Edinburgh University Press), 4.
104. See J. Goldstein, A. Freud and A. J. Solnit, *Before the Best Interests of the Child* (1980, Yale University Press). See also their *Beyond the Best Interests of the Child* (1973, Yale University Press). Discussed by Dickens, op cit at 466 et seq.
105. MacKay, "Perceptions of the Children Bill and beyond" (1989) 139 New LJ 505 at 508 (Joseph Jackson Memorial Lecture).
106. In the sterilisation cases it is possible to see the courts begin to draw up criteria for the decision-maker, albeit that sometimes the judges do not always spell them out as clearly as they could. See *re F* supra, and the discussion by I. Kennedy, op cit at 400–6. See also *re X* [1991] NZLR 365 (Hillyer J) (listing 17 factors). See also Grubb and Pearl, op cit at 449–50.
107. See *re B* supra, *re C* supra, and *re J* supra.
108. As occurred in *re J*: see Grubb [1990] All ER Rev op cit at 182–8.
109. See especially the speech of Lord Goff in *re F* at 80 (an adult incompetent case). Discussed, Grubb and Pearl, "Sterilisation – courts and doctors as decision makers" [1989] CLJ 380.
110. So, in *re J*, while the court relied upon the opinion of the expert put before the court that non-treatment was in the "best interests" of the baby, unlike the earlier case of *re C*, the court was prepared to examine the reasoning of the expert and did not simply adopt it as they seemed to do in *re C*. See Grubb [1989] All ER Rev 200 at 207
111. (1944) 321 US 158 at 170 (US Sup Ct).
112. *Jehovah's Witnesses* v. *King County Hospital* (1968) 390 US 598 (US Sup Ct per curiam); affirming (1967) 278 F Supp 488. The US cases are discussed in J. Areen, P. King, J. Goldberg and A. Capron, *Law, Science and Medicine* (1984, Foundation Press) at 1223–4.
113. See also *re B (wardship: abortion)* [1991] 2 FLR 426 (abortion authorised over mother's religious objection); *in re Eric B* (1987) 189 Cal App 3d 996 (Christian Scientist parents).
114. See also *Custody of Minor* (1979) 393 NE 2d 836 (Mass Sup Jud Ct)

(parents' consent to use of ineffective treatment (laetrile) for child with leukaemia amounted to neglect); contrast *re Hofbauer* (1979) 393 NE 2d 1009 (NY CA) (opposite conclusion but medical evidence against the use of laetrile was not so strong).

115. *re Phillip B* (1979) 156 Cal Rptr 48 (Cal CA) (Down's syndrome child aged 11 with IQ of about 60. Parents' refusal to consent to operation to correct congenital heart defect upheld even though his life would be shortened and health would progressively deteriorate). Quaere whether this case would have been decided the same in England (see *re B*, supra)?
116. See I. Kennedy, op cit ch. 5. This was also the common law in Scotland for "minors" i.e. boys aged between 14 and 18 and girls aged between 12 and 18. It was unclear whether "pupils", i.e. children below these ages, could consent if they had sufficient understanding: see D. W. Meyers, *The Human Body and the Law* (2nd edn 1990) at 156–8. The position in Scotland is now governed by section 2(4) of the Age of Legal Capacity (Scotland) Act 1991 which provides that a person under 16 (whether "minor" or "pupil") may consent to medical treatment if "in the opinion of a qualified medical practitioner attending him, he is capable of understanding the nature and possible consequences of the procedure or treatment". Notice, the statutory phrase "in the opinion of" seems to sanction a subjective test. This is probably not the position at common law; see I. Kennedy and A. Grubb, op cit at 215.
117. See I. Kennedy and A. Grubb, op cit at 180–215.
118. See Law Commission Consultation Paper 119 op cit, paras 2.14–2.31.
119. E.g. *Hunter* v. *Edney* (1885) 10 PD 93.
120. E.g. *Banks* v. *Goodfellow* (1870) 39 LR 5 QB 549.
121. E.g. *in re Beaney* [1978] 2 All ER 595.
122. E.g. *R* v. *Dunning* [1965] Crim LR 372.
123. On the relevance of "rationality" see *Sidaway* v. *Governers of Bethlem Royal Hospital* supra, per Lord Templeman at 509. *Lane* v. *Candura* (1978) 376 NE 2d 1232 (Mass App Ct) (irrational 77-year-old patient refusing amputation of gangrenous leg held competent to refuse treatment because she appreciated the nature and consequences of her decision). See also *re Quackenbush* (1978) 383 A2d 785 (NY). On the relevance of "reasonableness" see *Smith* v. *Auckland Hospital Board* [1965] NZLR 191 at 219 per Gresson J; *Hopp* v. *Lepp* (1979) 98 DLR (3d) 464 at 470 per Prowse JA.
124. Of course, some individuals may be incompetent to make any decisions, for example the unconscious or those in a comatose state.
125. See, for example, *Gillick* supra, per Lord Fraser at 409; per Lord Templeman at 432. See also *In the Estate of Park* [1954] P 112

(sufficient understanding to contract a marriage but not make a will).

126. [1991] 4 All ER 177. For a comment on the case see Bainham, "The judge and the competent minor" (1992) 108 LQR 194.
127. Supra at 183.
128. Supra at 187.
129. See *State of Tennessee* v. *Northern* (1978) 563 SW 2d 197 (Tenn CA) especially Drowota J (concurring); (72-year-old requiring surgical removal of gangrenous feet to save her life. Held incompetent to refuse surgery on basis she denied her condition and need for treatment).
130. Supra at 187.
131. Supra at 192.
132. Ibid.
133. This must be what Staughton LJ meant when he said that he agreed with Waite J that "the court can authorise medication, consistently with ... [*Gillick*] ... even if it has no greater powers than a parent" (at 188).
134. See P. D. G. Skegg, *Law, Medicine and Ethics* (1984) at 56–7.
135. [1972] Fam 302.
136. See *Hart* v. *O'Connor* [1985] AC 1000. See also L. Gostin, *Mental Health Services: Law and Practice* para. 26.26. Only if the other contracting party is aware of the mentally disordered person's incompetence will the contract not be binding, ibid.
137. See *Birkin* v. *Wing* (1980) 63 LT 80 and *Matthews* v. *Baxter* (1873) LR 8 Ex 132.
138. Only patients who are "liable to be detained" (but not all) fall within Part IV (s. 56). Similarly, Part IV does not apply to treatment that is not for the mental disorder. The legality of that is a matter for the common law; see L. Gostin, op cit at paras 20.10–20.16.5.
139. Included by Statutory Instrument. See, The Mental Health (Hospital, Guardianship and Consent to Treatment) Regulations 1983 (SI 1983 No 893), Regulation 16(1).
140. Section 57(2)(a). This seems to embody the common law concept of competence and consent; see *R* v. *Mental Health Act Commission ex parte W* (1988) *The Times*, 27 May.
141. Ibid Regulation 16(2).
142. See EL(90) P/85 and appended "Code of Practice – Mental Health Act" issued pursuant to section 118 of the Mental Health Act 1983.
143. Section 2 (for assessment); section 3 (for treatment); section 4 (emergency admission).
144. See L. Gostin op cit, paras 20.17–20.28.
145. Section 3(2).
146. Sections 63 and 58(1)(b).
147. Urgent treatment could have been given under section 62(1)(d)

(not irreversible or hazardous treatment necessary to prevent the patient behaving violently or being a danger to himself or others).

148. See *C* v. *Wren* (1987) 35 DLR (4th) 419 (Alberta CA) (16-year-old girl competent to consent to an abortion against the wishes of her mother).

149. See, for example, Eekelaar, "The emergence of children's rights" (1986) 6 OJLS 161 at 177–82.

150. *Department of Health & Community Services (NT)* v. *JWB and SMB* (1992) 66 ALJR 300 at 340. McHugh J (obiter) expressed the view that *re R* was wrong in this respect. The majority of the Court (Mason CJ, Dawson, Toohey and Gaudron JJ) referred to Lord Donaldson's judgment in *re R* but seemed neither to approve or disapprove of it (ibid at 305). Deane J also suggested that there might be a transitional stage in the intellectual development of a child where the authority to decide was shared between parents and child (ibid at 330). Brennan J (alone of the seven Justices) even cast doubt upon *Gillick* itself, remarking that it may have given insufficient weight to the "primacy of parental responsibility" (ibid at 324).

151. On the issue of confidentiality see Grubb and Pearl, "Medicine, health, the family and the law" (1986) 16 Fam Law 227 at 240. See also I. Kennedy, op cit at 111–17. For a different view see Montgomery, "Confidentiality and the immature minor" [1987] Fam Law 101.

152. In most cases, the parents' powers will not directly be before the court since, by definition, the court will be concerned (as in *re R* itself) with the scope of its own powers. Nevertheless, in *re J (a minor)* (1992), *The Times*, 15 May, Thorpe J agreed with Lord Donaldson's view.

153. The consent could also be given by anyone with "parental responsibility" under the Children Act 1989 or by someone who has temporary care of the child to the extent that it would be "reasonable in all the circumstances ... for the purpose of safeguarding or promoting the child's welfare" (s. 3(5)).

154. Supra at 186.

155. See supra at 184 and his earlier view in *Re J (a minor)*, supra. This is, of course, subject to the law of negligence. A doctor might be liable for damages for harm caused if he unreasonably fails to act on the parents' consent or, and this is important, *if he unreasonably acts in the face of the child's refusal.*

156. Supra at 184.

157. Supra at 423.

158. Supra at 185 (emphasis in original).

159. Supra text to notes 69–75.

160. Could this be one explanation of Lord Fraser's well-known five requirements (supra at 413)? Namely, that these factors are relevant

in determining whether the doctor is under a duty to treat the child once consent has been obtained.

161. See, for example, supra at 432 per Lord Templeman: "The parent is not bound by the infant's wishes".
162. Supra at 188–9.
163. Further, section 8(3) which provides that "Nothing in this section shall be construed as making ineffective any consent which would have been effective if this section had not been enacted", refers to the law relating to children under 16 years of age, in particular the view that competent children under 16 may consent to treatment. Therefore, it has nothing to do with retaining "parental rights" to consent. See *Gillick* per Lord Fraser at 408: "sub-s(3) leaves open the question whether consent by a minor under the age of 16 would have been effective if [section 8] had not been enacted".
164. See Report of the Committee on the Age of Majority (Cmnd 3342) (1967) under the chairmanship of Latey J (paras 474–84). Notice the contemporary commentary to section 8 in *Current Law Statutes Annotated* where the possibility of parental consent for a child patient under 18 who refuses treatment is mooted.
165. See the views in *Gillick* of Lord Fraser at 408 and Lord Scarman at 419 and Lord Bridge at 428 (agreeing with Lord Fraser and Scarman).
166. Supra at 185.
167. See *re F* supra, in which the House of Lords was anxious to avoid any conflict between a doctor's duty to an incompetent adult patient and his ability to treat without the patient's consent. See per Lord Brandon at 55–6. Cf. Lord Goff at 77–8.
168. See I. Kennedy and A. Grubb, op cit at 215.
169. See Bainham, "The judge and the competent minor" (1992) 108 LQR 194 at 198.
170. *F* v. *Wirral MBC* [1991] Fam 69.
171. See *Gillick* supra, per Lord Templeman at 434.
172. See Eekelaar, "The eclipse of parental rights" (1986) 102 LQR 4 at 8 and Eekelaar, "The emergence of children's rights" (1986) 6 OJLS 161 at 181 (arguing court could not). Cf. Bainham, "The balance of power in family decisions" [1986] CLJ 262 at 274–5; A. Bainham, *Children, Parents and the State* (1988) at 123–9.
173. See *J* v. *C* [1970] AC 668.
174. See *Re C (a minor) (wardship: medical treatment) (No. 2)* [1989] 2 All ER 791.
175. In *Department of Health & Community Services (NT)* v. *JMB and SMB* supra, Brennan J described this option as "erroneous in law and disturbing in its social implications" (at 325).
176. *Re P (a minor) (1981)* [1986] 1 FLR 272 (Butler-Sloss J) (abortion and IUD); *re G-U (a minor) (wardship)* [1984] FLR 811 (Balcombe

J) (abortion); *re B (a minor) (wardship: abortion)* [1991] 2 FLR 426 (Hollis J) (abortion).

177. See also *Department of Health & Community Services (NT)* v. *JWB and SMB* (1992) 66 ALJR 300, where the Australian High Court held that the Commonwealth Family Court had jurisdiction to authorise a sterilisation on a mentally handicapped 14-year-old girl in certain circumstances. A majority of the court (Mason CJ, Dawson, Toohey and Gaudron JJ) reached this conclusion even though they held that the parents of the girl did not have that power. The minority (Brennan, Deane and McHugh JJ) held that the parents had such a power also.
178. Supra at 186.
179. See *re J (a minor) (refusal of medical treatment)* (1992) *The Times*, 15 May, where Thorpe J, in exercising the court's inherent jurisdiction, authorised treatment on a competent 16-year-old girl who was anorexic and refusing treatment.
180. Supra at 189 and 192 respectively.
181. See the views of Thorpe J in *re J (a minor)* supra note 179.
182. *Re P* (minors) (wardship) (1992) *The Times*, 11 May.
183. But notice that the court cannot make a "section 8 order" once a child has reached 16 or which is made earlier but which will extend beyond his sixteenth birthday unless the case is "exceptional" (s. 9(6) and (7)).
184. Section 31.
185. Section 43.
186. Section 44.
187. Schedule 3 paras 4(1) and (4).
188. Schedule 3 paras 5(1) and (5).
189. For a similar provision in relation to "emergency protection order" see section 44(7), and for "interim care orders" see section 38(6).
190. On whether the court could *order* treatment see Grubb [1990] All ER Rev 182 at 188. The Court of Appeal held in *re J (medical treatment)* (1992) *The Times*, 12 June, that the court could not order a doctor to treat a patient contrary to the doctor's clinical judgment of what was in the "best interests" of the patient.
191. See *re J (medical treatment)* (1992) *The Times*, 12 June.
192. See the *parens patriae* power (not defunct) over adults who were of unsound mind: *re F (mental patient: sterilisation)* [1990] 2 AC 1 (HL).
193. Court of Appeal, 10th July 1992 (Lord Donaldson MR, Balcombe LJ and Nolan LJ); sub nom *re J* (*a minor*) (*refusal of medical treatment*) supra note 179.
194. See Dresser, "Feeding the hungry artist: legal issues in treating anorexia nervosa" (1984) *Wisconsin Law Review* 297 (discussing the

background to the condition and the legal issues).

195. See H. Bruch, *The Golden Cage: The Enigma of Anorexia Nervosa* (1979) at ix.
196. See the discussion in Dresser, supra note 194 at 302–309.
197. Devotees of popular music will recall that Karen Carpenter, who with her brother Richard made up the very successful singing duo, The Carpenters, tragically died of a heart attack in 1983 at the age of 32 having suffered from anorexia nervosa.
198. The Court of Appeal reaffirmed that the court had an inherent jurisdiction that could be exercised without the machinery of wardship. Lord Donaldson MR remarked that "the only additional effect of a child being a ward of court stems from its status as such and not the inherent jurisdiction . . . no 'important' or 'major' step in the ward's life can be taken without [the court's] consent". For a discussion see note 77.
199. Referred to at note 179.
200. See also Balcombe LJ: "[I]f [refusal of food] continued she would probably die; if it were not shortly reversed she would be likely to suffer permanent damage to her brain and reproductive organs."
201. [1975] Fam 47 at 61.
202. As regards children under 16, the court (rightly) confirmed that the House of Lords in *Gillick* had not been concerned with the court's powers.
203. At one point in his judgment Lord Donaldson MR stated that section 8 created an "irrebuttable" or "conclusive presumption" of competence to consent. Of course, it does no such thing. The concept of *Gillick*-competence, as it seems to have become known, is relevant to all persons whether adult or child. Section 8(1) merely puts the child aged 16 or over in the same position as an adult. Both are legally presumed to the capacity to understand sufficiently (and therefore be competent) to consent to medical treatment. But this presumption can in an individual case be rebutted by evidence of mental incapacity through mental illness, senility, physical injury or otherwise.
204. See Hoggett, "The royal prerogative in relation to the mentally disordered: resurrection, resuscitation, or rejection?" in MDA Freeman (ed.), *Medicine, Ethics and the Law* (1988: Stevens) at 85.
205. Court of Appeal, 30 July 1992 (Lord Donaldson MR and Balcombe and Butler-Sloss LJJ).
206. The case concerned an adult who refused a blood transfusion and then lapsed into unconsciousness. While accepting her right to refuse the blood transfusion (even in anticipation of unconsciousness) the Court of Appeal held that T had acted under the influence of her mother who was a Jehovah's Witness. The decision was not, therefore, really T's. Further, the judges accepted that T had not intended her decision to apply if her life were threatened. For a

discussion of this case, see Grubb, "Refusal of treatment: I – the competent adult" (1992) 3(1) *Dispatches* 1.

207. See *re J* (*a minor*) (*medical treatment*) (1992) *The Times*, 12 June, where the Court of Appeal refused to order a doctor to treat a seriouslly ill baby against his clinical judgment. While recognising that the court had the jurisdiction to do so, Lord Donaldson MR stated "I have to say I cannot at present conceive of any circumstances in which [to order a doctor to treat against his clinical judgment] would be other than an abuse of power . . .". Balcombe LJ stated that ". . . I can conceive of no situation where it would be a proper exercise of the [inherent] jurisdiction to make . . . an order . . . that is to order a doctor, whether directly or indirectly, to treat a child in a manner contrary to his or her clinical judgment".

208. See *in re X* (*a minor*) [1975] Fam 47 (public interest in freedom of information limited court's power).

209. *A* v. *Liverpool CC* [1982] AC 363 (court should not use wardship powers to supervise local authority's care powers conferred by statute).

210. There is a common law power temporarily to detain (and, perhaps, treat) mentally ill individuals but this is restricted to those who are an immediate danger to others and the mental health legislation has (impliedly) removed this judge-made power except where the detainer is a private individual: see, *B* v. *Forsey* 1988 SLT 572 (HL Scot). For a discussion, see L. Gostin, *Mental Health Services—Law and Practice* (1986, Shaw & Sons) at paragraph 21.11.

211. See the Mental Health Act 1983, discussed supra, 57–59.

212. Lord Donaldson MR may have had in mind the argument that enforced eating would not be treating W's mental illness as is required under the Act. However, treating the manifestation of the illness would help to alleviate the underlying illness itself and this is, almost certainly, covered by the treatment provisions of the Act, see: *R* v. *Mental Health Act Commision ex parte W* (1988) *The Times* May 26 (DC). Discussed by Fennell, "Sexual suppressants and the Mental Health Act" [1988] Crim LR 660.

213. See further PDG Skegg, *Law, Medicine and Ethics* (1984, Oxford University Press) at 115 (discussing the patient who suffers from kidney failure and whose ability to make a treatment decision is affected by his condition).

214. Lord Donaldson MR expressly reserved the position of the pregnant woman refusing life-sustaining treatment which would result in the death of her viable fetus. For a discussion of this, see I. Kennedy and A. Grubb, *Medical Law: Text and Materials* (1989) at 355–364. But contrast now the remarkable decision of Stephen Brown P in *res* (1992) *Independent*, 14 October.

215. Section 8 applies only to "surgical, medical or dental *treatment*" or

"diagnosis" (my emphasis) and so does not apply to non-therapeutic procedures such as organ or blood donation (per Lord Donaldson MR). Nor does section 8 cover the taking of a blood sample which is dealt with in section 21 (per Nolan LJ).

216. It is not linguistically impossible to construe a provision such as section 8 referring to "consent" to include "refusal"; see in *re Smith* (1972) 295 A2d 238 (Md CA) (construing a minor consent statute to prevent a child from having an abortion). See also the discussion in Dresser, supra note 194 at 366–373. See also, *In the Matter of Mary P* (1981) 444 NYS 2d 545 (abortion) and *Melville* v. *Sabbatino* (1973) 313 A2d 886 (mental health treatment).
217. For the only dissent that I know of, see Samuels, "Can a minor (under 16) consent to a medical operation?" [1983] 13 *Family Law* 30.
218. Lord Donaldson MR did, at least, cite the criticisms of his views in *Re R* but one is left with the impression that he had in mind the famous words of Mandy Rice-Davies at the trial of Stephen Ward: "[They] would say that, wouldn't [they]?".
219. Remember, of course, Lord Bridge expressly agreed with Lord Scarman.

Autonomy in the company of others

Susan Jinnett-Sack

Mainstream moral philosophy generally views humans as rational autonomous creatures exercising their will in the world to make decisions which are primarily self-regarding (affecting no person other than themselves in any morally cognisable sense). This model, when adopted by political philosophy and applied in the fields of law and biomedical ethics, has provided a powerful tool for elevating and protecting individual decision-making. However, this rights-based analysis is less useful in two situations: when issues arise which involve individuals who arguably do not fit the rational person model, and/or when issues affect third parties as well as the decision-maker (hereinafter referred to as "blended decisions").

The view of humans as purely rational autonomous creatures requires us to view the irrational in every person as an exception to the general rule of rationality. It also requires us to view the irrational person as the exception. Alternative views of man's essential nature from such diverse sources as classical philosophy, Christian thought and the re-examination of classical philosopy by such philosophers as Iris Murdoch and Bernard Williams do not view such behaviour as anomalous, but as definitional of our humanity. These alternative views lead to different concepts of moral decision-making from the mainstream view.

Part I of this chapter will explore these alternative views of what it is to be human in light of evaluating the applicability of

Choices and Decisions in Health Care. Edited by A. Grubb.

the resulting moral philosophy to people as they actually are. Part II will examine the implications of the differing philosophical views of people's nature for moral decision-making. It will contrast a will-centred model with motion as the central metaphor to one which focuses on vision as the appropriate metaphor. Part III will examine the tension between Mill's and the common law's views of liberty and individual responsibility and the blended decision scenario.

The playing out of these theoretical models in the public realm through law (primarily the doctrine of State interest in the United States and public policy in England) in relation to withdrawing medical treatment and compulsory pre-natal treatment will be discussed in Part IV.

I. A moral philosophy should be inhabited[1]

The rational man

It is beyond the scope and skill of this chapter to critique Kantian philosophy's model of human nature and its role in moral decision-making. However, taking as its line of thought the idea of "inhabiting" a moral philosophy, it would be useful to briefly examine the type of person that emerges from Kant's philosophy.[2]

Kant does not see man as solely a creature of rationality, but he does locate man's worth as a person in his moral self, exemplified by his rational aspect.[3] He takes as one of his primary assumptions that man's characteristics have developed to further the goal toward which they are best suited. The human desire for mere happiness is seen as ancillary to the goal of having a good will, in and of itself. Happiness cannot be the true goal of man for two reasons. First, because the result would have been more readily achieved by having man governed by instinct alone, and second, because reason would be irrelevant since it does not, in his view, further mere happiness.

> "For since reason is not sufficiently serviceable for guiding the will safely as regards its object and the satisfaction of all our needs (which it in part even multiplies) – a purpose for which an implanted natural instinct would have led us much more surely . . . its true function must be to produce a will which is good, not as a means to some further end, but in itself; and for this function reason was absolutely necessary in a world where nature, in distri-

> buting her aptitudes, has everywhere else gone to work in a purposive manner."[4]

Kant goes on in this passage to discuss a role for the good will that sets it in counterweight, almost of necessity, to the idea of a more daily type of happiness. He appears to relegate the joys of a life lived within the context of family, work, home, community to a lesser form of thinking, the mere sensible, and dwell on a plane which "... can even reduce happiness to less than zero without nature proceeding contrary to its purpose ...".[5] The true contentment in life is in fulfilling a purpose which is determined by reason alone, even if this goes against one's natural inclinations.

Kant's moral framework is one which compels us to fulfil a duty to the highest-order good, reason, and not to do so because of a desire for the consequences. Thus, an act is good because of the principle that it embodies, and because of our adherence to that principle and not because of any ulterior motive. The principle which is to guide us in all actions is the concept of the universal law or Categorical Imperative. A summary description of this principle is that:

> "A rational being must always regard himself as making laws in a kingdom of ends which is possible through freedom of the will – whether it be as member or as head."[6]

The image that emerges from Kant's beliefs reduces the morally significant, as well as active, aspect of man to his rational self as expressed through his will. Moral good arises when one acts, not from inclination, but from moral duty. All other aspects appear to be ones which must be controlled and which generally only interfere with and cloud our judgment as we seek to determine the good. The good must be universalisable, with the necessary corollary that all rational beings must count equally as ends and not as means to be used to achieve another's goals.

As will be discussed further below, this aspect of Kant's work is echoed in the liberal political philosophy of such writers as John Stuart Mill. Kant's emphasis on the essential equality of individuals and the need to further one's own goals only to the extent that one could advocate their furtherance by all provided a structure whereby great extensions of political liberty could be justified. However, Kant's philosophy can also be seen as highly procedural in focus. Kant posits man in a certain form (reason acting on will in the moral sphere), states rules (Categorical Imperative) and good results. It is unclear, however, how reason alone was to provide sufficient guidance to the question of how one is to live one's life.

One could argue that Kant's image of man as the rational individual acting out of moral duty on principles of universal applicability was reinterpreted in later political philosophy to keep the man but remove the duty. John Stuart Mill's *On Liberty* continues the emphasis on reason acting on the will as the defining aspect of what it is to be human. However, because his agenda was a political one, rather than a purely philosophical one, he used that argument to further a thesis that the ultimate good which each of us seeks is to be defined only by each of us. As such, the good that must be protected universally is the ability to seek one's own good individually. What has become universal is not the duty to achieve a good will, but the duty not to interfere with another's will. As such, far from condemning a desire to live like the South Sea Islanders as Kant did,[7] Mill would protect to the hilt our right to don grass skirts in January. Happiness in everday life has become a legitimate goal.

> "The only freedom which deserves the name is that of pursuing our own good in our own way, so long as we do not attempt to deprive others of theirs or impede their efforts to obtain it. Each is the proper guardian of his own health, whether bodily or mental and spiritual."[8]

Mill's philosophy looks to achieve the greatest happiness for individuals through allowing them the greatest freedom to pursue it as they see it. Mill's philosophy is inhabited by people much more motivated by concerns that are familiar to us: to be happy, to act out of desire, not duty, to do admittedly foolish things. At first reading, Mill presupposes rationality but does not require it, for he is not asking anyone to aspire to more than a negative restraint: to leave others alone. However, the limitation of his approach lies in his reliance on autonomy as the highest good to be protected to generate the greatest happiness, with little consideration of non-autonomous situations or individuals. Mill's view of society envisions many islands with only voluntary connections of a basically rational nature. As will be discussed further below, his emphasis on liberty falters when this isolation disappears.

The benighted creature

> "We are not isolated free choosers, monarchs of all we survey, but benighted creatures sunk in a reality whose nature we are constantly and overwhelmingly tempted to deform by fantasy."[9]

This altogether less sanguine view of human nature, as developed in the work of Iris Murdoch, Stanley Hauerwas and others, starkly challenges the rational autonomous man described above. In fact, one of the primary "fantasies" chosen in Murdoch's essays is Kant's view of man as a creature of reason driven to seek an external rational good. This desire for a perfect and necessary form and order is described as the philosopher's escape. More ordinary mortals escape through stories and beliefs which seek to impose a pattern on their lives and explain away the true chanciness and pain inherent in their existence.[10]

In Murdoch's view, to see the will as the irreducible carrier of moral value is to overestimate the power people actually have to choose. Their power is limited by several factors: their ability to see things for what they are; the actual availability of choices; and the presence of external forces. The greatest difficulty for true moral understanding is man's ego: his inability to see another for what it is without putting himself in the centre of the analysis.

The view of man as solitary, imminently educable and capable of self-knowledge is described by Murdoch as the happy marriage of Kant (minus his metaphysical background), utilitarianism and modern psychology.[11] It is the prevalent view today in liberal political theory, philosophy and biomedical ethics. It is inherently optimistic. Without diminishing its value in that arena, Murdoch reminds us of Hume's comment that we may be totally free and responsible politically but not in fact (alternatively that good political philosophy is not necessarily good moral philosophy).[12]

Murdoch does not dismiss the possibility of man achieving any moral good, in spite of her view that we are essentially fallible creatures. She does, however, believe that the moral life is achieved by very different means than the rationalists would use. This is the topic of part II below.

The ancient modern man

A recent re-examination of the relevance of classical thought to modern moral philosophy by Bernard Williams presents a way of viewing man that avoids the perceived extremes discussed above.[13] While speaking in very general terms, classical thought viewed man as having a disposition toward moral thought that was embodied in certain virtues. These virtues were more than mere habit, but were internalised dispositions of action, desire and feeling. It required the use of judgment on the part of the actor, a form of practical reason. It was through the exercise of these virtues that man achieves a life of well-being (Williams' translation of the term eudemonia).

The classical view of man saw him as an inherently moral creature who, through the exercise of internalised virtues, would try to achieve his own well-being. Well-being was not defined solely as the satisfaction of materialistic or transient desires, for a virtuous person would take satisfaction from such acts as helping others. Also, man was seen as a social individual whose role was to live a public as well as a private good. In contrast to the Kantian model which appears to depersonalise each of us to come up with a universalisable set of goals, the classical view looks to each person to find a personal well-being, having universalised the tools (the virtues) but not the goals.

II. Motion versus vision

The view of human nature which philosophers hold necessarily leads to differing concepts of the nature of moral decision-making. Only if one has an idea as to how one believes such decisions are made can one address perceived failures or limitations in that process.

The rational decision

Kant's view of man appears to generate only one way to make moral decisions. One's actions are not considered in terms of consequences *per se*, but of the principle represented. The situation was to be stripped of its uniqueness, down to its generic characteristics, and then it was to be universalised. The question must be asked if all people, faced with this situation, should behave as I propose to do. If the answer was that this would lead to a desirable result (with little apparent guidance as to how one judged if the result was desirable other than to follow one's reason), then the choice was clear.

Kant's examples tend to either the simplistic (borrowing with no intention of repaying the money) or to the more complex (committing suicide), but resolved through an appeal, not to reason in and of itself, but to definite assumptions as to what is right.[14] In the suicide example, it is viewed as wrong because of a perceived inconsistency with the role of self-love to further life. Yet one could universalise a situation in which suicide was permissible when life offered more evil than pleasure and still have a society that could function and which fit Kant's other apparent views of a moral one. Its impermissibility can only really be established by reference to an independent sense of the inherent "wrongness" of suicide.

The significance of the Kantian view of moral decision-making historically has been to:

1. focus analysis on the generic aspects of a problem and eliminate any consideration of unique or extenuating circumstances;
2. legitimate the requirement for only one principle that can apply to all situations;
3. elevate reason to the level of the sole tool for decision-making.

We are then left with a system or moral decision-making that is rule based, highly legalistic, yet lacking in the law's acknowledgement of the significance of certain factual patterns. The procedure can address life's major mishaps, but not its daily decisions. This is in part because the guidance provided is for the individual to *do* something, for the will to act. Once the essentially theological backdrop is removed from this system, as it has been today, there is little clear guidance as to the goal towards which the will is to move an individual. Again, there may have been no intention on the part of Kant or his followers to set forth a moral philosophy that was accessible for daily life. However, to the extent that one accepts the thesis that moral philosophy has humans as its intended object and not some alternative spiritual beings, and so long as humans live their life in the context of their daily lives, this difficulty has relevance.

The free decision

Once one moves to the essentially utilitarian outlook of Mill, the nature of moral decision-making has become both private and clearly goal-oriented towards the individual's self-defined happiness. Mill, for both personal as well as political reasons, was intensely interested in protecting personal lives from the intrusions of others. So here we do have a focus on recognisable human lives, but the guidance which is given is to leave everyone alone, so long as harm is not being caused to another. Social coercion, whereby people were prevented from doing what they believed right by peer pressure, was of great concern to Mill. Homogeneity of thought was anathema.

It should be stressed that Mill, in *On Liberty*, was writing political, and not moral, philosophy and as such there is no distinct attempt to develop an idea of what is a moral good in an affirmative sense. Instead, the focus is on what is required for individuals to be put in a position so they are free to seek their own good, be that in Christianity, humanism, snake-handling or enlightened self-interest.

> "There is no reason that all human existence should be constructed on some one or some small number of patterns. If a person possesses any tolerable amount of common sense and experience, his own mode of laying out his existence is the best, not because it is the best in itself, but because it is his own mode."[15]

The interaction between Mill's universal principle, and the areas of public acts affecting others, immorality and purely self-regarding acts, is not as clear cut as the rest of his philosophy. It is to this area that part III will address itself.

To see a thing clearly

> "Modern moral philosophers have failed to understand that moral behavior is an affair not primarily of choice but of vision. They see all moral agents as inhabiting the same world of facts; thus they discriminate between the different types of morality only in terms of acts and choices. But differences of moral vision or perspective may also exist."[16]

In contrast to the Kantian model which looks to single formulas and rational argument, there is an alternative view of moral decision-making which sees not motion of the will, but vision by the soul, as the core of moral decision-making. Borrowing from Simone Weil, Murdoch uses the concept of "attention" to describe moral thought. Attention is the "... idea of a just and loving gaze directed upon an individual reality."[17] It is in the constant attempt to see things for what they are, and not for what we wish them to be that moral choices are made and growth occurs. By focusing only upon the moment of choice, Murdoch believes that most modern moral philosophy has lost contact with the importance of the internal dialogue which we all hold with ourselves about our world and how we are to live.

Referring to the philosophical debate on the reality of inner versus outwardly perceived thoughts, Murdoch argues that there is moral significance to those changes of thought which, in our everyday speech, we would refer to as a "change of heart". By ignoring that progress, philosophers exaggerate the importance of the public *act* of choosing and diminish the importance of the private work of moral thought.

> "But if we consider what the work of attention is like, how continuously it goes on, and how imperceptibly it builds up structures of value round about us, we shall not be surprised that at crucial moments of choice most of the business of choosing is already over. This does not imply that we are not free, certainly not. But it implies that the exercise of our freedom is a small piecemeal business which goes on all the time and not a grandiose leaping about unimpeded at important moments . . . What happens in between choices is indeed what is crucial."[18]

Far from dealing with the proverbial alternative spiritual being, Murdoch equates virtue with reality, believing that the ability to see things as they really are to be the most difficult task humans have. The skill that must be developed to act morally is the ability to see a reality other than ourselves: "the non-violent apprehension of differences".[19] In this view of moral decision-making, the necessary characteristic for each of us to exercise our freedom is not will, but humility. Humility is used by Murdoch as the concept that links freedom with moral thought, for by humility she means:

> "not a peculiar habit of self-effacement, rather like having an inaudible voice, [but] it is selfless respect for reality and one of the most difficult and central of all virtues."[20]

The emphasis on the quality of one's daily life and thoughts and the necessity to strive to develop the necessary virtues for moral life links Murdoch strongly with the classical philosophers, particularly Aristotle. Her use of the concept of the good as an explicit goal for moral thought, in contrast to freedom or autonomy, distinguishes her sharply from modern mainstream moral philosophy. While she denies any belief in God or an existence for man outside of his allotted time on earth, her description of the good and its uses closely corresponds to a concept of God, minus the institutional theology. For that reason, theologians such as Stanley Hauerwas have explored her philosophy for its contribution to the idea of vision in moral development.

The connection between Murdoch's view of man as a "benighted creature mired in fantasy" and her view of moral development through attention to reality is that she sees the task as an exceptionally difficult one that few of us will either identify accurately or achieve. Discipline and focus are required to develop the necessary moral imagination and moral effort. The work to be done is necessarily private and progresses in infinitely tiny steps.

III. The limits of self

The limits of Mill's liberty

Moral philosophy would be much simpler if we were all rational friendless orphans without dependants. Analyses could proceed based on considerations of autonomy, self versus other regarding decisions, freedom and rights. Most people, being rational, as well as autonomous, would be considering the ramifications of their decisions and acting as they saw best to further their own good. All foolish and even harmful decisions would be respected as expressive of one's individuality and autonomy, so long as one did not cross the line into "incompetence". The world would then fit Mill's description of boundaries between protected private and scrutinised public action:

> "But there is a sphere of action in which society, as distinguished from the individual, has, if any, only an indirect interest: comprehending all that portion of a person's life and conduct which affects only himself or, if it also affects others, only with their free, voluntary, and undeceived consent and participation."[21]

Yet even Mill acknowledges that there are situations, short of intended harm to a third party (which are addressed by the criminal law's sanctions), in which an act's effects sufficiently impinge on a third party or on society so as to fall outside the realm of protected liberty:

> "Whenever, in short, there is a definite damage, or a definite risk of damage, either to an individual or to the public, the case is taken out of the province of liberty and placed in that of morality or law."[22]

Mill admits of two categories under which society may interfere with individual action: if that action renders a person unable to fulfil a prior obligation or represents a breach of duty of if the action results in a perceptible harm to another. These two categories represent a significant exception to Mill's general theories of liberty, but they appear to have received little critical examination, either by Mill or by his commentators.

Examples of Mill's exceptions include a man whose drunkenness prevents him from supporting his family or a policeman who is drunk on duty and, therefore, unable to discharge his obligations to the public. He carefully emphasises throughout these discussions that is is not the conduct *per se* that law or morality may seek to punish or enjoin. Instead, it is the breach of obligation and/or duty.[23]

While this approach seeks to preserve the purity of his belief that individual conduct not be subject to restraint, in practice it is a distinction without nearly the great difference he may have supposed. As mentioned at the beginning of this section, most people's destructive conduct in some way breaches an obligation if only because most adults have families for whom they are responsible. Most adults have jobs whose performance one could argue was an obligation if there was any public reliance upon it. Thus, it begins to appear as though the exception to the rule engulfs the rule when analysed in terms of numbers in each category.[24]

An alternative explanation for the apparently large exception to Mill's idea of liberty is that he did intend such a result. Mill was writing a political and social treatise at a time when his ideas were quite radical (as some of their implications still are today). However, one could argue that his system includes both rights *and* obligations and that he in no way intended to disavow certain generally accepted moral and legal obligations of his time. Thus, he wanted to establish one's right to a private life of whatever kind one wanted, but within certain limits. Those limits, however, appear to have been more significant than is sometimes attributed to him.

Mill's philosophy can be analysed both in terms of a public versus a private sphere of action, where the latter is protected from interference or as a self-regarding versus other-regarding distinction where the purely self-regarding action is protected. By positing the rule in favour of liberty and against societal intervention so strongly, with the exceptions somewhat in the "footnotes" so to speak, these exceptions have not received the analysis that they would require. It is easy to leave the solitary homeless man drunk in the park when he *is* viewed as isolated than when he is viewed as the absent supporter of dependent children. Note that Mill would not prevent society's interfering in that case, seeing his behaviour as a breach of his obligations to his family.[25] Note also that most commentators today would argue that Mill supported their belief that it is unjustified paternalism by society to interfere in such a case.[26]

Self versus other: legal limits

To view the "harm to others" principle as the sole goal of the criminal law is not only a radical view, but also is not the view that the law takes in the United States or England. The criminal law can be organised by categories of harm: harm to others; offence to others; harm to self; and harmless wrongdoing.[27] The vast bulk of the criminal law addresses itself to the clear-cut cases of harm to others: murder, robbery, rape, assault. Offence to others is the more obscure category of deeply offensive conduct that society has criminalised because of their near-universal moral offence (such as desecration of dead bodies). Harm to self reflects those areas where society has historically criminalised acts such as suicide and prize fighting out of a belief that in no case is such an act beneficial or one which we wish to protect for other reasons. Harmless wrongdoing is generally viewed as an example of legal moralism since its examples tend to lack "victims" in the traditional sense and it seeks to prevent "voluntary" acts.

This schema for viewing the law has been outlined because it is significant for seeing how the law tries to deal with cases where the harm to one, while clearly the primary harm, does not stop there but extends to another. The critical decision is to determine when that "spillover" becomes of a nature that the criminal law should take notice of it. Feinberg's very thoughtful legal philosophy in this area, as well as his stature in the field, makes it worth while to examine how he addresses such situations.

Feinberg's treatise has as an explicit goal the defence of a liberal interpretation of the law such that the principle of harm to others is the limit to the criminal law, with limited exceptions only under the other categories.[28] His viewpoint closely parallels Mill's:

> "... respect for a person's autonomy is respect for his unfettered voluntary choice as the sole rightful determinant of his actions *except where the interests of others need protection from him*."[29]

> "*When interests of third parties are not involved*, every person's moral right to govern himself surely outweighs the "right" of benevolent intermeddlers to manipulate him for his own advantage, whether that advantage be health, wealth, contentment, or freedom. If there is such a thing as personal sovereignty, even the subsequent increase in a person's freedom is no reason for invading his domain without his consent."[30]

Feinberg's language has been quoted at length to make two points. First, that the abhorrence with which Feinberg and most liberal thinkers view perceived instances of paternalism in the law leads them to discount instances in which the only way to prevent harm to a third party may be to interfere with someone with the intent of benefiting both, but also to avoid harm to the third party. This discounting occurs by not considering the harm to the third party actionable, rather than by re-examining their limitations on "interference".

The second point is the caveat that one's liberty stops at the beginning of another person's liberty is a given, but one that is still philosophically relegated to the exception. Again, politically this may make sense but even Feinberg spends little time addressing the possibility that far more actions are self *and* other-regarding than clearly one or the other. He writes that:

> "We can assume, therefore, that in some societies, at least, and at some times, a line can be drawn (as Mill claimed it could in Victorian England) between other-regarding behavior and conduct that is primarily and directly self-regarding and only indirectly and remotely, therefore trivially, other-regarding. If this assumption is false, then there is no interesting problem concerning legal paternalism, and certainly no practical legislative problem, since all "paternalistic" restrictions, in that case, could be

> defended as necessary to protect persons other than those restricted, and hence would not be (wholly) paternalistic."[31]

It is not the intent here to claim the equal and opposite extreme view that there are no actions that are inherently immune from review, but that the "assumption" that Mill, Feinberg and others make is too weighted in the direction of self-regarding by disregarding the reality of human relationships.

One of Feinberg's most intriguing paragraphs is one addressing the possibility of a society that is not so clearly divided between self and others and in which the balance is not so overwhelmingly individualistic.

> "... imagine a beleaguered garrison of settlers under attack from warlike Indians. Everyone is working furiously to repel the assault ... At the peak of the excitement, John Wayne becomes so bored and depressed, that he withdraws with the announced intention of killing himself. 'After all,' he says, 'my life is my own and what I do with it is my own business.' Of course, he could not be more wrong. What he does is everybody else's business since the issue is so close that the withdrawal of one party threatens to tip the balance. There is no distinction in these circumstances between self-regarding and other-regarding, or between not helping and positively harming."[32]

Feinberg concludes that insofar as any more complex society comes to resemble a garrison situation, any debate over legal paternalism becomes "otiose". He quite interestingly goes on to use a less fantastical illustration, in which he states that while one person's primarily self-regarding act of becoming a drug addict may be tolerated, when a significant enough percentage of people in a community take this path, then the principle of harm to others comes into play. Then, he says, this is a case where taking action against the individuals can be done purely under the harm-to-others principle.[33] It takes only a step, and not even a jump, to see the relevance of that description, and not Mill's to much of American society today.

While legal philosophers, such as Feinberg, have been enlarging the concept of self for the purpose of restricting societal standing to regulate, legislators have in many instances been moving in the other direction, though oft-times straining to find a rationale other than legal paternalism. Examples range from helmet and seat-belt laws, to restrictions on tobacco and liquor advertising.[34]

It is not the point in this thesis to examine in depth the various rationales that are used to justify legislation that on its face appears paternalistic. It is to note that there is a serious tension between our avowed insistence on individual responsibility and autonomy, and the concrete actions we take in insisting that certain actions are too irrational to allow individuals to do with societal approval. Note that these are actions which we do not generally believe one would be "incompetent", in the medical or legal sense, to want to do, but merely irrational.

IV. The State at the bedside

When one enters the area of the law relating to medical decision-making, there does appear a potential counterweight to the liberty principle discussed above. Whether it is termed "public policy" in England or "State's interest" in the United States, the concept is similar. The law recognises certain situations in which society has the right to assert that its interests be considered in balance with the individual's. It arises in medical cases where we believe that a person is incapable of protecting their own interests and/or when the person we rely upon to protect their interest is not doing so (an extension of the *parens patriae* doctrine) and in situations where the State believes the proposed course of conduct may violate an important public policy, regardless of the individual's competence. The role of the State's interest in medical treatment cases will be examined here for the purpose of determining the utility of expanding its role to address other situations where an individual's perceived autonomy rights come into conflict with another's well-being.

Withdrawal of medical treatment in the United States

The State's interest in medical treatment cases has been defined by courts in the United States to comprise four major concerns:

1. preservation of life;
2. prevention of suicide;
3. protection of third parties; and
4. protection of integrity of the medical profession

To the extent that suicide has been generally decriminalised in the

United States, category 2 has been subsumed into category 1, though this has tended to undermine the rationale of category 1 as an interest in withdrawal-of-treatment cases. Categories 1 and 3 are of most interest here and will be considered in depth below. Category 4 is not of relevance to the discussion here, as it arises primarily in cases considering active euthanasia and its effect on the role of the medical profession.[35]

Cruzan v. Director, Missouri Department of Health In the United States, the most recent authoritative discussion of the role of the State's interest in medical treatment cases was by the Supreme Court in *Cruzan* v. *Director, Missouri Department of Health*.[36] In that case, the court was considering the withdrawal of artificial food and hydration to an automobile accident victim, Nancy Cruzan, who, as a result of brain injury, was in a persistent vegetative state with no hope of recovery. Her family, as well as her court-appointed guardian, felt that not only was it in her best interest to do so, but that her prior expressed views on the matter supported their decision. While the trial court granted their request for an order permitting the withdrawal, the Supreme Court in Missouri reversed and there was an appeal to the Supreme Court.

The Supreme Court decided by a 5–4 majority that the State of Missouri was permitted by the Constitution to require "clear and convincing" evidence of an individual's desire to forgo life-sustaining treatment in a non-terminal, yet permanently incompetent state. This burden of proof did not violate Nancy Cruzan's Fourteenth Amendment liberty interest in avoiding unconsented medical treatment, though the court conceded this interest was fundamental. Further, the majority held that the State's interest in the preservation of life is a relevant State interest to assert in this context, and hence the State is not required to allow the substituted judgment of a family member in the absence of proof of the individual's wishes on the basis of "clear and convincing" evidence.

The majority opinion of Chief Justice Rehnquist reviewed the precedents concerning withdrawal of medical treatment, focusing on the line of cases in New Jersey beginning with the *Quinlan* decision, and continuing through *Conroy* to the trilogy of cases of *Farrell*, *Jobes* and *Peter*.[37] It noted that the standards adopted by the New Jersey Supreme Court in *Conroy* (a shifting standard of proof depending on the condition of the patient and the reliability of the evidence of their desires prior to incompetence) could be contrasted with the decision by the New York Court of Appeals in *O'Connor*, where the court refused to accept evidence of prior intent that was not "clear and convincing" and would not allow any family member to make the decision under a substituted judgment approach.[38]

The majority in *Cruzan* then used this broad review of differing standards to set the stage for a narrow definition of the issue in the case: does the Constitution prohibit Missouri's standard of evidence and its non-recognition of any other source of patient decision-making? The court first stated that the source of a right to refuse medical treatment does not derive from a constitutional right of privacy but from the Fourteenth Amendment's liberty interest. This is not surprising given the court's current conservative make-up and their desire for precedential reasons to limit any right of privacy so as to avoid expanding the grounds upon which, for example, their earlier abortion decisions can be supported.

Having established the right of the person to be protected, the court then stated that the legality of Missouri's action will depend on the interests which the State may validly seek to protect. Its reluctance to allow a "liberal" decision in this area (one which grants the widest discretion to individuals and their proxies) can be seen immediately, for the court asserts that the State interest in the protection and preservation of life make homicide and assisted suicide a crime (note the analogies selected) and that:

> "We do not think a State is required to remain neutral in the face of an informed and voluntary decision by a physically-able adult to starve to death."[39]

Since no one asked Missouri or the Supreme Court to do this, it is unclear what relevance this has, other than to indicate the direction the majority's decision was going to take. It does seem to indicate, however, that the majority views the State's interest in an individual to be broader than merely procedural and to encompass, in certain instances, intervention in situations where competent individuals make decisions against preservation of life.

However, the court was not presented with that broad a question and went on to say that in the face of that fact, Missouri was certainly permitted to impose a significant evidentiary burden, even though that shifted the presumption in any case against the party seeking to terminate treatment. Without going into the evidentiary arguments in depth, it is sufficient to say that the court used that burden to make an action of which they were fundamentally suspicious far more difficult to effect.

> "Finally, we think a State may properly decline to make judgments about the "quality" of life that a particular individual may enjoy, and *simply assert an unqualified interest in the preservation of human life to be weighed against the constitutionally protected interests of the individual.*"[40]

The court did not go into a legal or philosophical discussion of how those interests were furthered by the State's action in Nancy Cruzan's case. Since Nancy Cruzan was in a persistent vegetative state, this amounts to an assertion that the preservation of *mere* physical existence is sufficient grounds to allow the State to render difficult (the minority opinion argued impossible) the exercise of the rights that the court conceded that she still retained.[41]

The minority opinions, written by Justices Brennan and Stevens, differ from the majority's primarily in the weight given to the State's interest in the preservation of life in this situation. In Justice Brennan's opinion: "no State interest could outweigh the rights of an individual in Nancy Cruzan's position".[42] He goes on to assert that the State has "no legitimate general interest in someone's life, completely abstracted from the interest of the person living that life, that could outweigh the person's choice to avoid medical treatment".[43] Noting that even if he could theoretically conceive the State having such an interest, Missouri has by its other legislative acts demonstrated at best a "modest interest". He notes facetiously that Missouri has no law requiring everyone to seek medical treatment, nor any State insurance programme that would ensure medical treatment for all its citizens.

Justice Brennan does assert a role for the State, but it is the *parens patriae* role to determine that Nancy's best interests are met by a procedurally accurate and fair system. He distinguishes this from a procedure that will tend in almost all cases to thwart the wishes of individuals, since it is rare that oral evidence or any evidence short of a formal Living Will would meet the standards set forth by the Missouri Supreme Court. For him, a State does have an interest to fulfil here, but it is the *parens patriae* role which is not meant to be balanced *against* your wishes to counteract them, but to further them.[44]

Finally, both dissenting opinions would permit substitute decision-making in cases where it is not possible to determine clearly what choice the incompetent would have made for herself. Both feel that this is the only way to avoid a situation where the incompetent may have rights, but is totally barred from any effective exercise of them. Contrary to the majority, the minority opinion believes that it will be the exception where families do not act in the best interests of their member, and those cases are the kinds of cases that procedures can easily be designed to address. The majority has structured procedures as though all families were not only venal, but had some reason to act on it as well. Citing the New Jersey cases with approval, the minority notes that it is the family who has the closest idea of what the individual would view as her best interests, which should be the only concern and not some abstract idea that the State is interested in furthering. In a memorable turn of phrase, Justice Brennan writes:

> "In these unfortunate situations, the bodies and preferences and memories of the victims do not escheat to the State; nor does our Constitution permit the State or any other government to commandeer them.[45]

McKay v. Kenneth A. Bergstedt The first higher State court to consider a State's interest in this area since the Supreme Court's decision in *Cruzan* was the Supreme Court of Nevada in *McKay* v. *Kenneth A. Bergstedt*.[46] While the death of the plaintiff arguably rendered that case moot, the court rendered an opinion to establish guidelines for the withdrawal of medical treatment for non-terminal competent adults and in the process established a "fifth State's interest" in medical treatment cases.

Kenneth Bergstedt was a non-terminal competent adult quadriplegic who petitioned the court for an order permitting the removal of his respirator and the admission of sedatives (and absolving the individual who did so from liability) upon the impending death of his father and sole caretaker. He also requested a declaration absolving him of suicide in the removal of his life-support system. It should be noted, since the dissent in *Bergstedt* finds it of significance, that at the time of his petition the plaintiff had used his respirator for over 20 years, since an accident in a pool at the age of 10. His desire to remove it and die arose, and it was so conceded, from his fears as to his quality of life upon the death of his father (who apparently was the one who eventually removed the respirator for his son and entered a hospice and died himself two days later).

That the court's approach in *Bergstedt* differs fundamentally from the majority in *Cruzan* can be seen from its opening remarks.

> "One of the verities of human experience is that all life will eventually end in death ... It would appear, however, that ... prospects for slipping away during peaceful slumber are decreasing. And, for significant numbers of citizens like Kenneth, misfortune may rob life of much of its quality long before the onset of winter."[47]

After summarising the primary four interests that the State has that are to be weighed against the individual's rights in these cases, the court stated that there is a fifth concern of the State which is:

> "... in encouraging the charitable and humane care of those whose lives may be artificially extended under conditions which have the prospect of providing at least a modicum of quality living."[48]

The first significant difference between this court and the *Cruzan* court is the difference between an assertion that it is mere physical life that the State may preserve as opposed to a life with a certain quality of life. "[D]eath is a natural aspect of life that is not without value and dignity", the court stated and explicitly aligned itself with the New Jersey line of cases and not with the Missouri approach.[49]

The balancing of the State's interests in life and the individual's liberty interest in refusing medical treatment led the Nevada Supreme Court to conclude that, in situations involving competent adults who are irreversibly sustained by artificial life-support systems or some form of "heroic, radical medical treatment" and enduring physical and mental pain and suffering, the State's interest in the preservation of life will generally *not* outweigh the individual's right to decide on his own fate. In making this decision, the court stated that they attached great importance to Bergstedt's own assessment of his quality of life and his desire not to continue it. However, had he not died prior to the court's decision, the court would have required that the fifth interest it enunciated be fulfilled by assuring the court, essentially, that Kenneth Bergstedt's decision was an informed one, not clouded by fear of the unknown and ignorance over available support and medical assistance.

The Nevada Supreme Court carefully rejected Justice Scalia's position in *Cruzan*, and stated that in no way was Bergstedt's refusal to continue with the treatment he had begun the moral or legal equivalent of suicide. It is important to note for later discussion herein that the court distinguished his position from that of a healthy competent individual:

> "It is equally clear that if Kenneth had enjoyed sound physical health, but had viewed life as unbearably miserable because of his mental state, his liberty interest would provide no basis for asserting a right to terminate his life with or without the assistance of other persons."[50]

The court believed that the distinction which Justice Scalia failed to draw was the difference between:

> "Choosing a natural death summoned by an uninvited illness or calamity and deliberately seeking to terminate one's life by resorting to death-inducing measures unrelated to the natural process of dying."[51]

The Court stated clearly that the State's interest in preserving life related to preserving *meaningful* life. Contrary to the position in Missouri, that allowed Bergstedt to make the determination, subject to the limitation that he had crossed a stated objective threshold of injury/illness which, in effect, rendered his decision rational. Thus, the court used an objective threshold test to prevent the case supporting a right to commit suicide, but then a subjective standard took over that allows the individual to decide whether he wishes to refuse treatment.

The court in *Bergstedt* reluctantly set forth a procedure to be followed to facilitate the exercise of an individual's liberty interests when he is terminally ill or even if he is not. The reluctance arose because they strongly favoured extra-judicial procedures, but did not wish to leave individuals remediless until the Legislature acted. The court set forth a procedure which allowed a terminally ill patient's interest in self-determination to prevail over the State's interest in the preservation of life. In the case of non-terminal patients, however, the weighing of the

State's versus the individual's interests was to be determined by any district court judge on an expedited hearing basis.

It should be noted that a thoughtful dissent was filed in this case which argued that because there was no adversarial posture to the case (all parties, including the Attorney-General, desired the same result), there was no case in controversy and no opinion should have been rendered. The judge noted that this absence of controversy in the legal sense meant that no briefs had been argued in favour of not allowing what he believed was a court-sanctioned suicide to occur. The dissenting judge felt that it was quite significant that Bergstedt had lived for over 20 years in the state which he now felt was unbearable and that his situation was not clearly analogous to the "withdrawal" of medical treatment cases which the majority opinion used as precedent.

The dissenting opinion referred to a brief, which was filed too late to be considered legally, by the general counsel for the National Legal Center for the Medically Dependent and Disabled. This brief argued that, while withdrawal may be humane in the case of the near dead or irreversibly comatose, it is a different matter when the withdrawal of these items is "... admitted to be the immediate and proximate cause of the death of a person who concededly is seeking to take his own life".[52] The dissent argued that the ventilator should not be transformed into a heroic measure after 20 years, merely because the plaintiff's father was dying and he had not received any counselling or support which would assist him in coping with his situation. It should be noted that the majority would require just such counselling and it was only the intervening death of the plaintiff that made that point moot. The dissent was also concerned that the majority opinion would reinforce negative stereotypes of disabled citizens by allowing what amounts to a judicially sanctioned suicide only because the individual involved is disabled.

The purpose of this section is not to exhaustively review the case history in the United States relating to the exercise of the State's power to intervene to protect its interest in the preservation of life.[53] It was to make two points: first, that whether or not a court is going to allow the withdrawal of medical treatment, the State's power to bar any such action in the interest of the preservation of life is always explicitly preserved. The differences in approach by the courts exist at the level of the weight that such an interest is given in any particular fact situation.

Secondly, the analysis that is given of a State's interest in these cases is cursory and often conclusory. Nowhere is there a clear philosophical statement of the connection between the particular case and the State's interest short of stating that it is too obvious to need discussion. Although both *Cruzan*, and to a greater extent *Bergstedt*, explore an idea of harm to the community by allowing certain views of disability to prevail, there is no full exposition of these ideas.

Pre-natal treatment without consent in the United States

When we turn to the other arm of the State's interest doctrine that arises in medical treatment cases, the protection of innocent third parties, the courts are on easier ground analytically. The paradigm case for this doctrine is a pregnant, or recently delivered woman, typically a Jehovah's Witness, who is in need of a blood transfusion to save her life and/or the life of her fetus. While courts have reluctantly allowed Jehovah's Witnesses to refuse blood transfusions and die on the basis of their religious freedom, they have not allowed them to refuse transfusions for their already born children or, in the case of pregnancy, for the benefit of the fetus. The court steps in and, in exercise of its *parens patriae* power, orders the transfusion for the benefit of the fetus. The language of the New Jersey Supreme Court in *Raleigh Fitkin-Paul Morgan Memorial Hospital* v. *Anderson*[54] is typical:

> "... the welfare of the child and the mother are so intertwined and inseparable that it would be impracticable to attempt to distinguish between them with respect to the sundry factual patterns which may develop. The blood transfusions ... may be administered if necessary to save her life or the life of her child ..."[55]

When the factual pattern shifts, and the case involves a mother of an infant, the result has been the same, though the reliance on *parens patriae* is somewhat stronger since the court has to benefit the mother against her wishes to avoid the harm to the infant. This pattern presented itself in *President and Directors of Georgetown College*,[56] where the District of Columbia Circuit, the highest federal court to consider this issue, handed down its opinion through Judge Skelly Wright:

> "The patient, 25 years old, was the mother of a seven-month-old

> child. The State, as *parens patriae* will not allow a parent to abandon a child, and so it should not allow this most ultimate of voluntary abandonments. The patient had a responsibility to the community to care for her infant. Thus the people had an interest in preserving the life of this mother."[57]

An analysis of the Jehovah's Witnesses line of cases is less fruitful than might be imagined for exploring the limits of autonomy where third parties are involved. While these cases do preserve vitality for the doctrine that one's liberty interest – one's right to be left alone – has its limits, they do so in a situation where most of the courts that have considered the issue regarded the individual's decision as bordering on the irrational. While freedom of religion is taken quite seriously under constitutional law, there is still the lingering feeling that the basic irrationality of the tenet upon which the refusal is based is sufficiently odd that the court is desperate to find a way around it. However, these cases *are* significant for the springboard they have afforded to other decisions imposing more significant medical treatment upon a pregnant woman for the benefit of her and/or the fetus, but without her consent. It is to these cases that this discussion will now turn.

Again, there is a paradigm factual situation for the majority of the cases where the State has invoked its right to protect innocent third parties in imposing medical treatment.: the forced Caesarean. In 1981, the Supreme Court of Georgia in *Jefferson* v. *Griffin Spalding County Hospital Authority*[58] issued an order authorising a hospital to perform a Caesarean, and any necessary blood transfusion, on a woman who had refused consent. The evidence was that the chances of survival for both the mother and child were not better than 50% for the mother and less than 1% for the child without the intervention. The refusal of consent was stated to be based on religious beliefs, but not of any known or organised group.

The court stated that the life of the child and the mother were at that time inseparable and it was, therefore, appropriate to "infringe upon the wishes of the mother to the extent it is necessary to give the child an opportunity to live".[59] The legal basis for this action was that the child's viability entitled it to the protection of the Juvenile Court Code of Georgia. Under the terms of that code, the child, even though unborn, was deemed to be "without the proper parental care and subsistence necessary for his or her physical life and health". Temporary custody of the child was placed with the appropriate welfare agency and that agency was given authority to consent to the appropriate medical treatment on behalf of the child. Custody was declared to terminate upon the birth of the child.

The court stated that the State has an interest in the life of this "unborn, living being" and that the intrusion to the woman of requiring the Caesarean was outweighed by the duty of the State to "protect a living, unborn human being from meeting his or her death before being given the opportunity to live".[60] While the facts of the case would support an argument that the compelled medical treatment was in the best interests of both the mother and child (given the 50% chance of death for the mother without a Caesarean), the court appeared to base its decision solely on the interests of the unborn child.

The supporting opinions of two other judges in the case did, however, clarify that their generally great reluctance to order medical treatment against the wishes of a competent adult was, in this case, mitigated by the apparent need of the mother for the treatment as well as the child.[61] They did, however, emphasise that at the stage that the fetus becomes viable, the interests of the mother must be weighed against that of the child and that it was not within the rights of the woman, even her First Amendment rights, to indirectly or directly cause the death of the child.

The most recent court in the United States to consider the issue of forced Caesareans is the Court of Appeals for the District of Columbia in *re A. C.*[62] This case had a somewhat tortuous history given that the court handed down at different times two opinions: the first confirming the permissibility of forced Caesareans in certain circumstances and upholding the trial court, and then subsequently the final decision of the Court of Appeals vacating its original decision and stating that forced intervention was impermissible. The facts of the case were particularly poignant, yet in a sense presented the most clear-cut situation, *if* there ever is to be one, in which an enforced procedure could be allowed without (or against) the mother's consent.

The mother in *re A. C.* was in a terminal condition suffering from leukaemia and in the 26th week of her pregnancy. She had become almost comatose when the doctors approached her husband and family to obtain permission to perform an emergency Caesarean section in an attempt, albeit without much chance of success, of saving the life of the child. The facts are sketchy in all three courts' opinions as to whether the woman consented because she was delirious and made no consistent statement of intent or refusal of consent. Most commentators, however, have taken the case to be one where consent was, for all effective purposes, refused.[63]

In confirming the trial court's order permitting the Caesarean, the Court of Appeals, in its first decision,[64] argued from the initial principle that parents may not utilise even their First Amendment rights to refuse life-saving treatment for their children. The Jehovah's Witnesses line of cases were then cited as cases where this principle was extended to children yet unborn, but viable. Noting that this was clearly a case where the state's interest in protecting innocent third parties runs squarely up against the woman's right to bodily integrity, the court held that subordinating the woman's rights, in this case, was permissible. The court declined to apply the more limited principle that treatment could only be ordered if it would benefit a baby expected to be born alive, but would not significantly affect the health of the mother. Noting that the woman was not expected to live for more than a day or two longer, the court found that balancing the harms inflicted was in the baby's favour.

In a full hearing en banc almost three years later, the District of Columbia Court of Appeals vacated the lower court's decision and ordered that the case be remanded in line with the instructions in their opinion.[65] The court held that the decision of a competent patient to refuse medical treatment governs "in virtually all cases". In the absence of a competent patient, the court is to use a substituted judgment standard to decide what she would have wished done had she remained competent. After that analysis is completed, the court held that balancing the imputed decision with the state's interest in the preservation of life of the mother or the child is permissible. However, the court went on to volunteer in dicta:

> "We do not quite foreclose the possibility that a conflicting State interest may be so compelling that the patient's wishes must yield, but we anticipate that such cases will be extremely rare and truly exceptional. This is not such a case.
>
> Having said that, we go no further. We need not decide whether, or in what circumstances, the State's interests can ever prevail over the interests of a pregnant patient. We emphasize, nevertheless,

> that it would be an extraordinary case indeed in which a Court might ever be justified in overriding the patient's wishes and authorizing a major surgical procedure such as a caesarean section."[66]

The court dismissed summarily the line of cases invoking a state's interest in the protection of third parties in exactly the factual situation presented in *re A. C.* Interestingly, there was no real discussion of the position of the child, as either a party to be considered or even in factual terms as to the consequences to it if the refusal of the Caesarean section was upheld by the court. While the court could have come to the same conclusion, the absence of any explicit acknowledgement of this aspect of their decision detracts from its intellectual honesty.

In so holding, the court distinguished in *re A. C.* an earlier decision in *re Madyun*[67] in which the trial court had ordered a Caesarean to be performed over the refusal of consent of a competent patient. In *re A. C.*, the court distinguished this case factually, stating that where the Caesarean was clearly of benefit to both the mother and the child, that the baby was at full term and the mother had been in labour for two days, and that *re Madyun* was not a case of conflicting interest of mother and fetus in medical terms. By contrast, they saw *re A. C.* as a case where the pregnancy was only in its 26th week, labour had not started and the Caesarean was not of benefit to the mother.

The court in *re Madyun* found that the State had frequently exercised its rights under the *parens patriae* doctrine as regards unborn infants at the state at which they were viable. Citing *Roe* v. *Wade*,[68] the court noted that in the third trimester the viability of the infant justified "unduly burdensome State interference with the woman's constitutionally protected privacy interest". In permitting the operation to go ahead, the court stated that:

> "All that stood between the Madyun fetus and its independent existence, separate from its mother, was, put simply, a doctor's scalpel. In these circumstances, the life of the infant inside its mother's womb was entitled to be protected ... It is one thing for an adult to gamble with nature regarding his or her own life; it is quite another when the gamble involves the life or death of an unborn infant."[69]

Citing *Prince* v. *Massachusetts*,[70] the court noted that it believed the religious beliefs of the parents, to the extent they supported their refusal of consent, no more entitled them to martyr the unborn viable child than it would one who was already born. It should be noted that in the court's opinion in *re Madyun*, contrary to the view taken of it in *re A. C.*, there was no discussion of benefit to the mother. In fact, the order of the court in *re Madyun* stated that given the significant risks to the fetus versus the minimal risks to the mother, the Caesarean was to be performed.

An opinion concurring in the result was filed in *re A. C.* by Judge Belson. However, he strongly dissented from the very limited – one could say non-existent – role that the state's interest in the preservation of life and innocent third parties played in the decision of the majority. Judge Belson felt that the trial court had clearly found A. C. to be incompetent and that it was not a reversible error for the trial court to have failed to apply a substituted judgment standard (as defined by the majority) when there was no precedent for such an approach in a case of this sort in any jurisdiction. No one in the family or at hand at the time of the trial court's decision had made a request to make a decision on A. C.'s behalf. Most significantly, Judge Belson pointed out that the statement by the majority that this was not a case where the State's interest in protecting the life of the unborn child would override the mother's interest was mere dicta since the majority of the court felt A. C. would have consented had she been competent. Thus, the majority view as to the role of the state's interest was not necessary to the decision. Most importantly, Judge Belson disagreed with the court's statement that the state, in effect, has no interest to weigh against that of the putative mother's:

> "I would hold that in those instances, fortunately rare, in which the viable unborn child's interest in living and the State's parallel interest in protecting human life come into conflict with the mother's decision to forego a procedure such as a caesarean section, a balancing should be struck in which the unborn child's and the State's interest are entitled to substantial weight."[71]

Judge Belson quite accurately stated that the majority's characterisation of the issue at hand as "the method of delivery" is an over-simplification at best, given that the choice of method virtually ensured whether the child died or had a chance to live. He went on to outline a balancing approach that would take into account the likelihood of survival of the child, the possible adverse effects on the woman's health and any relevant religious beliefs. He noted that he would find it legally justifiable to find that pregnant women who carried fetuses that had reached the stage of viability were a unique class of persons and were to be treated differently as regards their right to make decisions during pregnancy.

Withdrawal of medical treatment in England

For what would appear to be cultural, as well as legal, reasons there is no body of comparable English law to that in the United States regarding the extent of one's ability to request the withdrawal of life-sustaining medical treatment. To the extent that English medical practice defines its standards in terms of a "generally accepted professional standard", there has always been less room for individual opinion and disagreement. To the extent that the courts are not utilised to address these societal issues as pervasively as they are in the United States, there is an overwhelming likelihood that resolutions are achieved informally both within the profession and the family involved.

Common law in England allows a competent individual to decline treatment under the same general principle in the United States, that consent to a touching is required to avoid its being a battery.[72] While the doctrine of "informed consent" in its American sense has not been accepted generally, there is a growing trend to encourage that more information be given to patients and that the medical profession not be the sole determiners of what patients should be told. Thus, in *Sidaway* v. *Board of Governors of the Bethlem Royal Hospital*,[73] the leading case on this point, Lord Bridge specifically rejected the doctrine of *Canterbury* v. *Spence*[74] and stated that the doctor's duty of care in the area of medical disclosure was to be decided on the basis of expert medical evidence. He did, however, admit that "the judge in certain circumstances might come to the conclusion that disclosure of a particular risk was so obviously necessary . . . that no reasonably prudent medical man would fail to make it."[75]

To the extent that a competent person wishes to refuse life-sustaining treatment, England also has only had one reported instance involving a Jehovah's Witness. In *R* v. *Blaue*,[76] although not a medical treatment case, the court did not suggest that the doctor there would have been authorised to override a refusal to accept a blood transfusion by the decedent on religious grounds. Commentators have also stated that it is English law that one has the right to refuse to receive life-sustaining treatment, although as in the United States the statement is not made categorically.[77] For example, Professor Skegg notes that

> "*For the most part* doctors should not administer even life-saving treatment if the patient refuses consent and no one else is authorised to give it" [emphasis added].[78]

One assumes that the final reference is to cases of minority or cases where the court exercises its *parens patriae* power.

When one looks for cases such as Nancy Cruzan's and Kenneth Bergstedt's, there appear to be no English precedents. It is the opinion of some legal commentators, such as Kennedy and Grubb, that the English courts, if faced with such cases, would follow the approach of the American courts such as the New Jersey line of cases beginning with *Conroy* and the Massachusetts case of *Superintendent of Belchertown* v. *Saikewicz*.[79] This is not to suggest that these cases are entirely consistent, but only that their approach to these decisions in utilising either a best interests or a substituted judgment analysis would represent the approach most sympathetic to the English common law. It would seem less likely, however, that an English court would entertain the legal fiction of substituted judgment for a person who was never competent, but would, instead, utilise a best interests standard as more consistent with their approach in wardship cases.[80]

Mason and McCall Smith have, however, stated that they believe that if an English court were faced with a situation such as that in *Bergstedt*, where an affirmative action was required by the doctor to enable the patient's wishes to be met, it would not be permitted if it was seen to violate professional standards of the medical profession, as defined by that profession.[81] Citing the New Jersey case of *Re Farrell*, they note the language therein that a patient does not have the right to "compel a health-care provider to violate generally accepted professional standards".[82] It should be noted, however, that the court in *re Farrell* allowed the discontinuation of a respirator for a competent woman with amyotrophic lateral sclerosis (ALS).

It does appear to be open to question whether an English court would order the discontinuance of life-sustaining treatment for a non-terminal competent patient, especially where that would require the physician to take affirmative acts to alleviate pain, etc.

While England does not have the developed doctrine of State interest to fall back on as a limiting principle in this area, the heightened respect which is accorded to medical opinion, together with the concept of public policy generally in the law, would allow a court to find such an action impermissible. For the present, it is likely to continue a matter of individual medical and personal decision and, as such, may differ from case to case.

Prenatal treatment without consent in England

English law is consistent with the majority of US jurisdictions in recognising a cause of action for injury to a fetus only if it should be born alive.[83] This has left the law in the curious position where the assailant is better off having killed the victim than injured it. It is the troubling moral and legal ramifications of this approach that have led some to search for an alternative view of the status of, at least, the viable fetus.

As a starting point, doctors in England are not criminally liable for aborting a viable fetus under recent changes to the abortion law.[84] However, in contrast to American law, which uses "viability" as the benchmark for attaching certain legal rights due to the Supreme Court's holding in *Roe* v. *Wade*, English law has traditionally looked to the standard of a child "capable of being born alive". One can argue that this standard sheds no more light than viability, since it gives no guidance as to whether "alive" can be in an assisted state or for how long one must be "alive".[85]

The significance of all this for the area of non-consensual pre-natal treatment is that the legal position of the fetus in England is, if anything, less certain than in the United States. There is not a clearly developed body of rights-oriented case law which can easily attach to the fetus (admittedly at the cost of certain apparently irreconcilable conflicts with the mother). Secondly, the Congenital Disabilities (Civil Liability) Act 1976 specifically provides that a child may not pursue a cause of action against its mother if she is the party who caused the injury by her negligent conduct (section 1(1)). This issue was considered by the Law Commission and it was decided to bar it for reasons of policy: damage to the parent/child relationship and possible usage as a weapon in matrimonial disputes.[86] The latter appears to be an evil that could have been addressed otherwise, especially considering the few cases that award custody to the father, but the former issue is a much more difficult one.

Given the express prohibition of causes of action against the mother and the absence of any case precedent such as *re A. C.* on forced prenatal intervention, it is questionable what result an English court would reach if faced with such a situation. Any attempt to have the patient found "temporarily incompetent", thus allowing the State to exercise its *parens patriae* power under the Mental Health Act, appears highly unlikely. A case which required counsel to establish some type of mental illness which manifests itself by its adverse effect on another entity (albeit not one with legal standing) and requires "treatment" for this other entity and not the so-called incompetent was not the intent of the Mental Health Act.[87]

Mason and McCall Smith have noted the inherent dilemma of accepting the fetus as a patient, as well as the mother, and suggest the possibility of deferring treatment, when possible, until the child is born.[88] However, to the extent that this causes avoidable harm to the child, the problem is not necessarily avoided by the delay. It merely sidesteps the issue of whether the fetus has sufficient interests to be protected that the doctor should attempt to intervene on its behalf to compel treatment of the mother.

When action by the mother prior to the child's birth involves criminal or other conduct rising to the level of child abuse, English courts are more sympathetic to State intervention under its *parens patriae* power. In the case of *D (a minor)* v. *Berkshire County Council*[89] a child was placed under care at birth upon a positive drug test of its mother. The court considered that it was significant that the alleged conduct pointed to a behaviour that could reasonably be expected to continue rather than a single event.

When faced with the issue of wardship attaching prior to the birth of a child, however, English courts have been unwilling to go so far. In *Re F (in utero)*,[90] the Court of Appeal refused to make a fetus a ward of court upon application of the authority that its mother was a street person and not providing appropriate pre-natal care or the likelihood of an appropriate birthplace. The court stated that no wardship could attach under the principles of *Paton* v. *British Pregnancy Advisory Service Trustees*[91] and *C.* v. *S.*[92] because the fetus had no legal standing until birth and that the exercise of wardship was incompatible with the mother's liberty interests. The court noted the US precedents in this area and stated quite clearly that it was a legislative matter for Parliament to state how and in what circumstances protection was to be extended to unborn children, taking account of appropriate protection for the mother as, for example, Parliament has done in the Mental Health Act 1983.

In the company of others

E. M. Forster once wrote that while "[d]eath destroys a man, the idea of death saves him". Although the nature of humanity renders death, not a right as some have termed it, but an inevitability, it remains critical that it should not be a mere by-product of a court's analysis. While the knowledge of death may save adults from endless procrastination during their lifetime, actual death is a mere end for an infant.

One difference between a *Cruzan* or a *Bergstedt* case and *re A. C.* lies, in part, in the willingness of the court to acknowledge the presence of an "other" who must be recognised, who is real. In *Cruzan* and *Bergstedt*, the humanity of those individuals was never questioned, yet the courts involved looked to a larger community than that to decide what freedom and what rights were appropriate for the patients. In *Cruzan*, whether one agrees with the majority or minority opinions, a view of persons that requires us to consider the family of which they are part, and the larger society within which they lived, can be seen. In the majority opinion, the court clearly subordinated the feelings and desires of both the patient and her family to its view of what was in the community's interest. This was conceded in Chief Justice Rehnquist's opinion. While his view of family involvement in these matters was that it was too inherently self-interested to be relied upon by a court, he at least acknowledged their involvement.

The court in *Bergstedt* emphasised the community's responsibility to provide support and care for individuals who through disease or injury are in need of extended care. Their view of the State's interest in this area serves to promote individual autonomy as well as community regard. It is laudable that they were willing to emphasise the need for community involvement and balance an analysis concerned with Bergstedt's rights as an individual with the enhancement possible by others. This is an example where a consideration of individuals as interconnected members of a community can serve not necessarily as a limitation, but as a reminder of its benefits.

By contrast, the majority opinion in *re A. C.*, regardless of the "correctness" of the outcome, viewed A. C. in isolation from any community (including apparently her family) and, most importantly, from the child she was carrying. To describe the issue at hand in *re A. C.* as merely "the selection of the method of delivery" is to demonstrate either an inability, or most likely an unwillingness, to state publicly the direct effect of the court's order. Judgments reached several years after the events occurred did not require the court to respond with its full humanity to the same extent as the trial court was required to do.

To view A.C.'s dilemma strictly in terms of a rights analysis, as the court did, is to lock oneself into an inherent conflict in which one right must triumph over the other. To "balance" rights is too often viewed as the unprincipled way out, the way that admits of a certain evil to avoid a greater one only due to lack of moral courage. And when we lack the certainty to proclaim one right as pre-eminent over another, we generally delegate the decision to a procedure that will ensure that some individual involved makes the decision. This, for example, has been the law's approach until recently in the area of selective non-treatment of neonates.[93] It is the approach recommended by the DC Court when they stated that they did not wish to see such cases again and hoped that they could be resolved internally within the hospital/patient setting.

The second limitation of the emphasis on rational rights analysis is that it emphasises, as it did in *re A. C.*, the rights of the plaintiff without raising any question of duties or obligations on her part. As in bridge, only another right could be thrown on the table to trump her autonomy and right to bodily integrity. Thus, it is not surprising that nowhere in the majority opinion is there mention of any obligation that A. C. might have, having chosen to carry the child to the point of viability. Nor is there any explicit statement acknowledging that the preservation of a philosophical principle of autonomy and the woman's right to bodily integrity, in the case where the woman would die within a few days no matter what is done, means that a child who would otherwise have a chance to live, will die. If one is going to trade A. C.'s principles for the child's death, surely the least that could be done is to explicitly state so?

The real irony of the emphasis of the court's sole emphasis on autonomy/bodily integrity as the sole criterion for judgment is its inconsistency with what most people would probably have seen as the best course of action here. It is rare, outside a court of law, for one to find people willing to trade off death for principles of independence and matters of consent. If this were not true, we would have more than just the Jehovah's Witnesses refusal cases. This is not to make light of the importance of those ideas, but only to say that in cases involving matters of death, people do not generally weigh only rational criteria about the various competing rights. If that were true, we would never see the level of sacrifice by parents for children, and by children for older parents with which we are all so aware. It is the very detachment which we so prize in the law that, in cases such as these, allow the divergence of law and a consideration of the moral good.

To return to an earlier idea:

> "We are not isolated free choosers, monarchs of all we survey, but benighted creatures sunk in a reality whose nature we are constantly and overwhelmingly tempted to deform by fantasy."[94]

It is the lawyer's necessary fantasy to make humans generic, with rights which are applied universally to those similarly situated. In lieu of that, they can elevate procedure to take the place of substance. Thus, autonomous decision-making becomes the only goal: not any independent good embodied in the decision or any independent exercise of virtue. The question *and* answer are sought in a minute linguistic analysis of the incoherent speech of a dying woman, rather than extended to an examination of where, if anywhere, some good can be salvaged from tragedy, some life in the face of inevitable death.

But, one may rightfully say, that is the best that the law can do. It is not appropriate that the law should provide moral content to an individual's decisions. This is to ignore, however, the extent to which the procedure determines the substance of the decision as it did in *re A. C.* In this regard, however, the law must not be held solely responsible for what is also a general societal view, especially in the United States. The desire and struggle for equal rights in the areas of civil law since the Second World War is a major part of American mythology. The tendency to see a rights-based analysis as a universal solution to society's problems thus becomes more understandable given its notable successes. The need for emphasising the independence of patients, their right to information and control over their treatment is not presented here as a minor one. What is argued is that only to focus on that ability is to ignore the difficult work that remains to be done.

What is lacking is the necessary public discussion of various ideas of private and public good that would enable each of us to make decisions with greater recognition of their effect on others. This is not to suggest that there is only one such idea. It is, however, to suggest that the limits of our reliance on a model of detached autonomy should be obvious when considering issues such as that raised in *re A.C.* or in *Bergstedt*. To the extent that the only public vocabulary we have developed is one where I insist on the testing of the dominance of my rights over yours, we should not expect non-litigious resolution or any sense of community good or of personal obligation.

The power of the State, as exemplified by the transatlantic doctrines of State's interest and public policy, reflect to an imperfect degree the view of their citizens. Given the lack of homogeneity of views, it is not surprising that any exercise of authority, or lack of it, is subject to controversy. However, for the law to abdicate its traditional power as *parens patriae* over those who cannot speak for themselves would be to confirm that we ultimately have no connection, one to the other. Bernard Williams has noted that, in the context of utilitarian politics, "benevolence gets credentials from sympathy and passes them on to paternalism".[95] That fear, however, must not be used as a reason to banish sympathy by refusing to see the actual and real lives confronted in our philosophies and by our laws.

Notes and references

1. Murdoch, "The idea of perfection" in *The Sovereignty of Good* (London: Routledge & Kegan Paul, 1970), at 47.
2. While it is arguable that this is far too literal and simplistic a usage of Kant's philosophical work, it seems to be necessary as a starting point if his moral philosophy is to have any relevance outside the theoretical realm.
3. I. Kant, *The Groundwork of the Metaphysics of Morals* (New York: Harper & Row, 1964).
4. Ibid at 64.
5. Ibid at 110.
6. Ibid at 101.
7. Ibid at 90.
8. J. S. Mill, *On Liberty* (London: Pelican Books, 1974) at 72.

9. Murdoch, "Against dryness", in S. Hauerwas and A. MacIntyre (eds.), *Revisions: Changing Perspectives in Moral Philosophy* (University of Notre Dame Press, 1983) at 49.
10. Ibid See also Murdoch, "The sovereignty of good over other concepts" in *The Sovereignty of Good*, supra note 1, at 103.
11. Murdoch, "Against dryness", supra note 9, at 44.
12. Murdoch, "The sovereignty of good over other concepts", supra note 10, at 81.
13. B. Williams, *Ethics and the Limits of Philosophy* (Cambridge: Harvard University Press, 1985).
14. I. Kant, *Groundwork of the Metaphysic of Morals*, supra note 3, at 89–91.
15. J. S. Mill, *On Liberty*, supra note 8, at 132.
16. S. Hauerwas (ed.), "Vision and virtue", in *Essays in Christian Ethical Reflection* (Notre Dame: University of Notre Dame Press, 1974) at 34.
17. Murdoch, "The idea of perfection", supra note 1, at 34.
18. Ibid at 37.
19. Hauerwas, "Vision and virtue", supra note 16, at 39.
20. Murdoch, "The sovereignty of good over other concepts", supra note 1, at 93.
21. J. S. Mill, *On Liberty*, supra note 8, at 71.
22. Ibid at 149.
23. Ibid at 148–9.
24. The irony of following Mill's position too literally is that we actually create a class of people who are morally expendable because of their complete lack of connectedness to other members of society. Arguably, these people are the ones most in need of support and assistance, yet a doctrine such as Mill's can be used as justification for what amounts to neglect and indifference. We can be scrupulous in our defence of the "right" of the homeless to remain on the street, yet not address our obligation to provide acceptable alternatives.
25. J. S. Mill, *On Liberty*, supra note 8, at 148–9.
26. See, for example, the discussion in part III-B below of Joel Feinberg's limitations on permissible interference by the State. Another example in the biomedical field is found in Charles Culver and Bernard Gert's influential book, *Philosophy in Medicine* (New York: Oxford University Press, 1982) in which they argue that:

    "... only the evils of death and serious bodily injury .. are sufficient to make it irrational for one not to prefer experiencing the evil of detention." (at 168.)

    In the context of their discussion, detention was used as the term for non-consensual medical treatment.
27. J. Feinberg, *The Moral Limits of the Criminal Law: Harm to Self* (New York: Oxford University Press, 1986), at ix.

28. Ibid at 3 and 14.
29. Ibid at 68 (emphasis added).
30. Ibid (emphasis added).
31. Ibid at 22.
32. Ibid.
33. Ibid at 23.
34. For a discussion of the tension between our paternalistic and libertarian desires and a consideration of the appropriateness of judicial versus legislative enactments in this area see Shapiro, "Courts, legislatures, and paternalism" (1988) 74 *Virginia Law Review* 519.
35. For a discussion of the role of the State's interest in withdrawal of medical treatment cases, focusing on the bsence of any underlying rationale by the courts for its application, see Peters, "The state's interest in the preservation of life: from Quinlan to Cruzan" (1989) 50 *Ohio State Law Journal* 8912. Note that this article was written before the Supreme Court handed down its decision in *Cruzan*.
36. 760 S.W.2d 408 (Sup Ct Mo. 1988), aff'd (1990) US, 110 S. Ct. 2841, 111 L Ed 2d 224.
37. *Re Karen Quinlan*, (1976) 355 A2d 647 (Sup Ct NJ) cert den sub nom *Garger* v. *New Jersey* (1976) 429 US 922; *Re Conroy* (1985) 486 A2d 1209 (Sup Ct NJ); (1987) *Re Peter* 529 A2d 419 (Sup Ct NJ); *Re Jobes* (1987) 529 A2d 434 (Sup Ct NJ); *Re Farrell* (1987) 529 A2d 404 (Sup Ct NJ).
38. *In re Westchester County Medical Center on behalf of O'Connor* (1988) 531 NE2d 607 (Ct App NY).
39. *Cruzan*, supra note 36, at 2852.
40. *Cruzan*, supra note 36, at 2853.
41. Justice O'Connor's concurring opinion reflects more an assertion of federalism and its principles than a deeply held suspicion of the whole concept of withdrawal of medical treatment and surrogate decision-making. She states that the court did not decide the question of whether it would have been unconstitutional for Missouri to refuse to implement the instructions of a properly named surrogate for medical decision-making. She quite explicitly suggests that this is a better route to go in these cases. Ibid at 2858.

    Little will be said of the somewhat idiosyncratic concurring opinion of Justice Scalia other than to note that he does address the issue of the link between a State's interest in the preservation of life and its interest in the prevention of suicide. The term "idiosyncratic" is used given his insistence that there exists no constitutional question at issue here at all and, secondly, that a withdrawal of medical treatment amounts in all cases to suicide if death results.
42. *Cruzan*, supra note 36, at 2869.
43. *Cruzan*, supra note 36, at 2870.
44. Note that Justice Brennan's argument can be seen as circular, since the majority would say that it is also the role of the *parens patriae*

doctrine to protect the incompetent against her or another's decisions that are not in her best interests. It is not clear to them that withdrawal of medical treatment is in her best interests. In a PVS case, this is a difficult argument to sustain, but it might be relevant as a principle in less dire circumstances where a withdrawal of treatment was requested.

45. *Cruzan*, supra note 36, at 2878.
46. (1990) 801 P2d 617 (Sup Ct Nev).
47. *Bergstedt*, ibid at 621.
48. *Bergstedt*, ibid at 621.
49. *Bergstedt*, ibid at 623.
50. *Bergstedt*, ibid at 625.
51. *Bergstedt*, ibid at 626.
52. *Bergstedt*, ibid at 634.
53. Dyke, "A matter of life and death: pregnancy clauses in Living Will statutes" (1990) 70 *Boston University Law Review* 867. K. Knopff, "Can a pregnant woman morally refuse fetal surgery?" (1991) 79 *California Law Review* 499. D. Mathieu, *Preventing Prenatal Harm* (1991) (Dordrecht: Kluwer Academic Publishers). T. Mayo, "Constitutionalizing the right to die" (1990) 49 *Maryland Law Review* 103. P. Peters, "The State's interest in the preservation of life: from Quinlan to Cruzan" (1989) 50 *Ohio Law State Journal* 8912. B. Robin-Vergeer, "The problem of the drug-exposed newborn: a return to principled intervention" (1990) 42 *Stanford Law Review* 745. D. Shapiro, "Courts, legislatures, and paternalism" (1988) 74 *Virginia Law Review* 519.
54. (1964) 201 A2d 537 (NJ Sup Ct) (per curiam), cert den (1964) 377 US 985.
55. *Raleigh Fitkin*, ibid at 538.
56. (1964) 331 F2d 1000 (DC Cir.) cert den (1964) 377 US 978.
57. *Georgetown University*, ibid at 1011.
58. (1981) 274 SE 2d 457 (Sup Ct Ga).
59. *Jefferson*, ibid at 457.
60. Ibid.
61. *Jefferson*, ibid at 461.
62. (1987) 533 A2d 611 (DC Sup Ct) aff'd (1988) 539 A2d 203 (Ct App DC), vacated (1990) 573 A2d 1235 (Ct App DC, en banc).
63. See, for example, K. Knopoff, supra note 53 at note 110.
64. (1988) 539 A2d 203 (Ct App DC).
65. (1990) 573 A2d 1235 (Ct App DC, en banc).
66. *In re AC*, ibid at 1252.
67. (1986) 114 Daily Wash L Rpt 2233 (DC Super Ct).
68. (1973) 410 U.S. 113.
69. *In re Madyun*, supra note 67.
70. (1944) 321 US 158 at 170.
71. *In re AC* supra note 65 at 1254.

72. [1988] Fam 52.
73. [1985] A.C. 871.
74. (1972) 464 F2d 772 (DC Cir).
75. I. Kennedy and A. Grubb, *Medical Law: Text and Materials* (London: Butterworth, 1989) at 1066.
76. [1975] 1 WLR 1411.
77. I. Kennedy and A. Grubb, supra note 75 at 1066.
78. P. D. G. Skegg, *Law, Ethics and Medicine* (Oxford: Oxford University Press, 1985) at 33 (emphasis added).
79. I. Kennedy and A. Grubb, supra note 75 at 1071.
80. See, for example, *Re D* [1976] Fam 185.
81. J. K. Mason and A. McCall Smith, *Law and Medical Ethics* (London: Butterworth, 3rd edn. 1991) at 334.
82. Ibid at 334.
83. Ibid at 139. Congenital Disabilities (Civil Liability) Act 1976. At common law, see *B* v. *Islington Health Authority* [1991] 1 All ER 825.
84. Mason and McCall Smith, supra note 81 at 114. See also Human Fertilisation and Embryology Act 1990, s. 37(4) amending Abortion Act 1967, s. 5(1).
85. Mason and McCall Smith, supra note 84. But see *Rance* v. *Mid-Downs Health Authority* [1991] 1 All ER 801.
86. Mason and McCall Smith, supra note 81 at 139.
87. *Re F (mental patient: sterilisation)* [1990] 2 AC1.
88. Mason and McCall Smith, supra note 81 at 141.
89. [1987] AC 317.
90. [1988] Fam 122.
91. [1979] QB 276.
92. [1988] QB 135.
93. Ibid.
94. See, for example, Schneider, "Rights discourse and neonatal euthanasia" (1988) 76 *California Law Review* 151.
95. Williams, supra note 13 at 89.

The persistent vegetative state: medical, ethical and legal issues

Bryan Jennett*

Many patients now survive acute episodes of damage to the brain that would previously have proved fatal. Although the effectiveness of modern resuscitation and intensive care enables some of these patients to make a good recovery, others are left with irrecoverable brain damage. Some of them regain consciousness but are mentally and physically disabled and may be dependent. A small number of them have permanently lost the function of the cerebral cortex – the grey matter, the thinking, feeling part of the brain. When we described the resulting clinical condition in 1972, Professor Plum and I proposed the term "persistent vegetative state".[1]

Clinical condition

These patients are sometimes loosely described as being in persistent or irrecoverable coma. However, the word coma strictly applies only to patients who are in a sleep-like state, whereas vegetative patients have long periods during which their eyes are

* Professor Jennett's chapter was delivered as a Lent Lecture and is an expanded version of a paper published in the *British Medical Journal* which is reproduced by kind permission (Jennett and Dyer, "Persistent vegetative state and the right to die: the US and Britain" (1991) 302 *British Medical Journal* 1256).

Choices and Decisions in Health Care. Edited by A. Grubb.

open. During that period they may reflexly turn their head and eyes towards a loud sound or a bright light, and may briefly follow a moving object. All four limbs are spastic and there is no voluntary movement, but the arms are able reflexly to withdraw from a painful stimulus. Reflex grasping and groping movements with the hands occur, the face may grimace, and groans and cries may be heard. Small amounts of food or fluid put in the mouth may be swallowed, but their survival depends on feeding through a tube into the stomach either through the mouth or through a small opening in the abdomen. Breathing is normal and they do not need a ventilator.

The wide range of reflex activity indicates continued function in the brain stem, which is a primitive part of the brain. There is, however, no evidence of any psychologically meaningful response, no sign of a working mind; these patients never utter a recognisable word nor obey commands. However, relatives and inexperienced professional observers may for a time interpret certain reflex activities as suggestive of meaningful responses, but careful observation over a period of time dispels any doubts. There are no readily available laboratory tests which can determine that the cerebral cortex is out of action. The modern radiological imaging techniques of computed tomography scanning and magnetic resonance imaging show only that there is severe damage to the brain, whilst the EEG records a wide range of different types of electrical activity, none of which is diagnostic of this state. Special research investigations of a small number of vegetative patients have shown that their consumption of oxygen in the brain is very low, similar to the level during deep anaesthesia.

Causes of the vegetative state

Severe head injury accounts for almost half the vegetative survivors after acute brain damage. The impact injury mechanically tears large numbers of fibres in the white matter of the brain that are going to, and coming from, the grey matter or cerebral cortex, which is therefore isolated. Another common cause is deprivation of oxygen to the cerebral cortex, when resuscitation after cardiac arrest is carried out too late to save the complex cerebral cortex, which is more sensitive to lack of oxygen than is the more primitive brain stem. Cardiac arrest is most often due to a heart attack or a medical accident under anaesthesia. Less common causes of acute brain damage leading to vegetative survival are hypoglycaemic attacks in young diabetics, and tumours or infections in the brain.

About ten new vegetative survivors per million of the population occur each year in the UK. Many die within the first year, usually as the result of pneumonia. However, more than half of those still alive at one year live for three years or more, and some survive for 10, 20 or even 30 years. Prolonged survival depends only on basic nursing care with the provision of adequate nutrition by gastric tube, and most patients are in long-term institutions or nursing homes. A few patients are vegetative for a few weeks after an acute insult and then make some degree of recovery, but no useful recovery is known to have occurred in patients who are still vegetative after three months.

Ethical issues

The prolonged survival of vegetative patients presents dilemmas for their families and carers as well as for society. These have attracted little public attention in Britain, but in the United States many families of vegetative patients have sought court rulings to discontinue life-sustaining treatment after hospitals had refused such requests. In more than 80 cases, spread across many States, the courts have supported the wishes of families, but the refusal of Missouri to follow these precedents brought the US Supreme Court its first "right to die" case in 1990.

There seem to be no self-regarding interests for the patient in having vegetative survival prolonged. Surveys among several different groups in more than one country indicate that most people consider that survival in the vegetative state is an outcome of illness or accident that is worse than death.[2] However, because the patient has lost the neurological mechanisms by which he could suffer either mental distress or pain, the burdens of prolonged survival fall on others. His family and friends have to witness the indignity of this state in someone they once knew, while health care staff know that they are engaged in a futile endeavour, and that this means that their skills are being denied to other patients who could benefit. However, the reasons commonly justifying withdrawal of life-sustaining measures do not apply because vegetative patients are neither suffering nor terminally ill, and they cannot express a wish to refuse treatment.

A consensus has nonetheless developed in the United States that it is ethically and legally appropriate to discontinue life-sustaining treatment for vegetative patients. This is probably related to the strength in that country of the informed consent movement, which aims to protect the rights of competent patients to refuse treatment, including that which may save or sustain life. This attitude is reflected in do-not-resuscitate orders and "living will" legislation, which was first introduced in California in 1976.[3] But there is concern there also that incompetent patients should not have their lives prolonged inappropriately. Declarations by the American Medical Association in 1986[4] and 1990[5] specify that treatment may properly be withdrawn from vegetative patients, and that this includes artificially provided nutrition and fluid. Many American courts have agreed with this principle, which the Supreme Court's recent decision confirmed. There is, however, still some debate about who should make this decision for an incompetent patient, and whether evidence is needed about the attitudes or wishes of that particular patient.

The case of Nancy Cruzan

Nancy Cruzan was 25 when she sustained a head injury in 1983 which left her in a vegetative state. In 1987 her parents requested the removal of the gastrostomy tube, to allow her to die. The hospital sought a legal ruling before allowing the doctors to do this, and in July 1988 a State court found in favour of the family"s request. The State Attorney-General appealed and the Missouri Supreme Court reversed the decision.[6] It maintained that the State had an unqualified interest in the preservation of life, and that treatment could be terminated only if there was clear and convincing evidence that Nancy would have refused such treatment. The State undertook to pay the medical expenses of continued survival, estimated at $130 000 per year.

The family appealed to the US Supreme Court, which heard oral argument on 5 December 1989. That same night doctors, lawyers, philosophers and clergy debated the case for two hours on public service television. In June 1990 the Supreme Court decided by 5 votes to 4 that constitutionally Missouri could require a high standard of evidence of Nancy's wishes before it allowed withdrawal of treatment.[7] In the event further witnesses came forward to testify that Nancy has expressed such wishes before her accident. In December 1990 the same Missouri State Court that had first heard her case ruled that feeding could be stopped. When she died 12 days later she had been vegetative for almost eight years, and her parents had petitioned various courts on eight occasions that she be allowed to die. During the last 12 days of her life, pro-life groups attempted to secure injunctions to restore feeding, but both State and federal courts refused to grant these.

The Supreme Court decision

In its first "right-to-die" case the US Supreme Court upheld the right of a competent patient to refuse treatment. Delivering the majority opinion on the *Cruzan* case Chief Justice William H. Rehnquist said: "Missouri may legitimately seek to safeguard the personal elements of this choice between life and death through the imposition of heightened evidentiary requirements."[8] He went on:

> "Close family members may have a strong feeling – a feeling not at all ignoble or unworthy, but not entirely disinterested either – that they do not wish to witness the continuation of the life of a loved one which they regard as hopeless, meaningless and even degrading. But there is no automatic assurance that the view of close family members will necessarily be the same as the patient's would have been, had she been confronted with the prospect of her situation while competent".[9]
>
> Dissenting, Justice Brennan said that Missouri was imposing "improperly biased procedural obstacles" in the way of the constitutional right to be free of unwanted medical treatment, which Stevens J (also dissenting) thought would limit the right to "those patients who had the foresight to make an unambiguous statement of their wishes while competent."[10]

Noting that the decision did not set new standards for medical practice, the *New England Journal of Medicine* was concerned by the almost complete lack of attention to medical reality, and that the professional and personal roles of the patient's physician were completely ignored.[11] An accompanying statement from 34 bioethicists was an attempt to prevent the kind of misrepresentation of the ruling that they felt might lead to serious adverse consequences for other hopelessly ill patients.[12] They urged physicians to encourage their patients to make an advance directive (living will), which is recognised by legislation in most US States, and which may also allow a person to appoint a family member or friend to make medical decisions for them (durable power of attorney). In the absence of such directives many State courts before *Cruzan* allowed feeding to be discontinued, relying on the family's judgment of what the patient would have wished. This was based on the constitutional right to privacy, which includes the right to decline life-prolonging treatments. Federal legislation introduced in November 1991 requires hospitals to inform all patients on admission of their right to make an advanced treatment declaration, or to appoint a proxy decision-maker.[13]

The position in Britain

There is no constitutional right to privacy and no legislation to underpin the use of living wills in Britain. A working party on living wills in 1987 concluded that English law would already require doctors to act according to a patient's previously expressed wishes.[14] However, to ensure that their decisions about treatment are respected, and are not overruled by doctors who think they know best, it recommended that patients in Britain, like those in America, should be able to rely on living wills or durable powers of attorney. Although these proposals have attracted considerable support[15] there has been no attempt to legislate. Recent changes to English and Scottish law provide for a power of attorney to remain in force even though the person who made it becomes imcompetent. But powers of attorney in Britain are limited to decisions about property and finance. Scots law, however, has a useful device which has recently been used more frequently for making decisions about incapacitated persons. On petition, the Court of Session can appoint a tutor dative, who may make decisions relating to welfare, which could include medical treatment. This device is recommended to its members by the Voluntary Euthanasia Society of Scotland, which issues a living will to its members. Outside of such specific arrangements, however, family members in Britain have no legal right to make treatment decisions for their relatives who are incompetent adults.

The issue of withdrawing life-sustaining treatment from vegetative patients has not so far reached the courts in Britain, leaving doctors and families in a legal vacuum. In practice, doctors often take decisions to discontinue treatment in consultation with families and without involving the courts. Like the American Medical Association, the British Medical Association accepts that patients can refuse treatment and that artificial feeding is regarded as treatment.[16] It is, however, uncertain whether English or Scottish courts would follow American courts in rejecting the suggestion that discontinuation of nutrition for a vegetative patient might constitute a criminal homicide. When a district coroner in England was consulted in 1989 by doctors proposing to do this for an accident victim, he is reported to have stated that he would have no choice but to refer the case for criminal investigation.[17] That case has subsequently been discussed at length on television and in the press, with the doctor and the father of the teenage patient both expressing concern at being unable to act in what they consider to be his best interest.[18] However, when the same question was asked of the Central Legal Office for the Scottish Health Boards it advised that the Procurator Fiscal service (which investigates suspected crimes in Scotland) would not consider such action inappropriate. It advised that a second medical opinion should be obtained and that the relatives should be consulted. But, the advice went on, the family should not be asked for their consent to withdrawing life-support. This is because in Scotland, as in England, relatives have no legal right to consent on behalf of an incompetent adult.

There is some parallel with the sterilisation of mentally handicapped women, a practice only recently challenged in the courts. In the case of *Re F*, the House of Lords ruled that the court could not consent to treatment but it could declare that it would not be unlawful.[19] The Law Lords relied on the common law doctrine of necessity, which allows the treatment of unconscious patients in their best interests. English and Scottish courts have traditionally been more inclined to adopt the "best interests" approach to taking decisions on behalf of another, rather than that of "substituted judgment" (trying to decide what the individual would have wished if competent). The difficulty with patients in the persistent vegetative state is that it might seem that to them life and death are the same, making it difficult to argue that death is in their best interest.

There has been little public discussion of this issue in Britain. Few would like to see the courts regularly involved in what most regard as clinical decisions, a view shared by most doctors and many judges in America.[20] Legislative backing for living wills and enduring powers of attorney for medical decisions could be helpful, but would provide only for the minority of persons who had chosen to make advance directives. The recent report from the Institute of Medical Ethics was intended to promote wider discussion between the public and medical professional bodies on whether the withdrawal of nutritional support is the appropriate way to deal with vegetative patients.[21] Certainly the matter has attracted considerable attention from the broadcast and print media. Moreover, discussion documents have been produced by the Law Commissions of both England[22] and Scotland[23] addressing the issue of decision-making for mentally incompetent adults. Although neither refers to the problem of vegetative patients the opportunity has been taken to draw this problem to their attention.

Notes and references

1. B. Jennett and F. Plum, "Persistent vegetative stage after brain damage: a syndrome in search of a name" (1972) i *Lancet* 734–7.
2. B. Jennett, "Vegetative state: causes, management, ethical dilemmas" (1991) 2 *Current Anaesthesia* 57–61.
3. Natural Death Act 1976 (Ca).
4. AMA Council on Ethical and Judicial Affairs "Withholding or withdrawing life-prolonging medical treatment" (1986) 236 *JAMA* 471.
5. AMA Council on Scientific Affairs; "Persistent vegetative state and the decision to withdraw or withhold life support" (1990) 263 *JAMA* 426–30.
6. *Cruzan* v. *Harman* (1988) 760 SW2d 408 (Sup. Ct Mo.).
7. *Cruzan* v. *Director, Missouri Department of Health* (1990) 111 L Ed 2d 224 (US Sup Ct).
8. Ibid at 243.
9. Ibid at 247.
10. Ibid at 257 and 280 respectively.
11. G. J. Annas, "Nancy Cruzan and the right to die" (1990) 323 *New England Journal of Medicine* 670–3.
12. 34 Bioethicists. Bioethicists' statement on the US Supreme Court's Cruzan decision (1990) 323 *New England Journal of Medicine* 686–7.
13. Patient Self-Determination Act 1991.
14. Centre of Medical Law and Ethics, King's College, London and Age Concern, *Living Wills: Consent to Treatment, Report of Working Party* (Edward Arnold, 1988).

15. Gillon, "Living wills, powers of attorney and medical practice" (1988) 14 *Journal of Medical Ethics* 59–60.
16. BMA Medical Ethics Committee: discussion paper on treatment of patients in persisent vegetative state. BMA, London 1992.
17. Brahams, "Euthanasia in the Netherlands" (1990) i *Lancet* 779–80.
18. "Son lost but not gone", *Sunday Times*, 28 April 1991 at 44–6.
19. *Re F (mental patient: sterilisation)* [1990] 2 AC 1.
20. Lo, Rouse and Dornbrand, "Family decision making on trial: who decides for incompetent patients" (1990) 322 *New England Journal of Medicine* 1228–32.
21. Institute of Medical Ethics Working Party: "Withdrawal of life-support from patients in a persistent vegetative state" (1991) 337 *Lancet* 96–8.
22. Law Commission Consultation Paper No. 119. *Mentally Incapacitated Adults and Decision-Making* (HMSO, London, 1991).
23. Scottish Law Commission, Discussion paper 94, *Mentally Disabled Adults: Legal Arrangements For Managing Their Welfare and Finances* (HMSO, Edinburgh, 1991).

Geriatric medicine: some ethical issues associated with its development

Margot Jefferys

This chapter has been prompted by thoughts raised by a project in which I am currently engaged. It is a study of the development of geriatric medicine as a medical specialty with recognition as such in the National Health Service (NHS). There were two principal objectives for the project.

The first was simply to obtain oral accounts from those involved in the early development of the specialty (i.e. in the 1940s and 1950s) who were still alive in 1991. These accounts will ultimately be lodged in the National Life Story Collection of the National Sound Archive – a part of the British Library which is the guardian of our cultural heritage. The second was to examine historical records of various kinds in order to understand the reasons why a formally recognised medical specialty of geriatrics developed in the UK and not in the main elsewhere.

The field of the medical care of individuals in old age bristles with issues which require consideration from an ethical point of view. Two which spring to mind at once are already the subject of much public debate and I shall consider them only briefly before raising others which have not had so much attention outside the confines of the medical profession itself.

Choices and Decisions in Health Care. Edited by A. Grubb.

Euthanasia

There is first the issue of euthanasia, which itself can be defined in two ways. It can be taking the procedures necessary to assist an individual who has expressed the desire to bring about the end of her or his own life before that event would occur "naturally", in which case it is generally given the prefix *voluntary*, or it can be the taking of active steps to hasten the end of life in individuals who appear to be suffering great pain or discomfort, without their specific consent but in circumstances where the professionals in whose care they have been placed believe such lives to be beyond amelioration. At present it is, strictly speaking, illegal either to assist an individual to hasten her or his own death or to undertake procedures which would have the same effect with or without the consent of the individual concerned. Nevertheless it is believed that both kinds of euthanasia are practised quite commonly by professionals involved with the care of the individuals concerned, because they are more likely than lay carers to have the knowledge and the access to the resources required to bring about the desired end. If, in the future, euthanasia in some form or other were to be legalised, members of the medical profession are likely to be nominated as the agents not only to carry out the euthanasia but also to determine the circumstances under which it would be considered legitimate and not an unjustifiable assault on an individual.

The moral issues are obviously complex. Where voluntary euthanasia (for example through the use of advance directives such as "living wills") is concerned, the right of individuals to determine their own futures, including the right to decide when their own life should end, is at stake; but also involved is the right of individuals who are needed to assist the patient to comply with the wish. Some doctors, as in the case of abortion, may have objections on religious or other conscientious grounds. Where patients are not able to express their own preference, the issues are even more complex.

While euthanasia is a general issue which could relate to individuals of any age – for example, to severely physically disabled or mentally distressed young adults – it is most likely to be contemplated by and for those who are nearing the end of a "natural" life span.[2] Hence it cannot be ignored as an issue affecting the everyday decisions which geriatric physicians and others giving professional care to old people may have to take.

Resuscitation

A closely related issue is that of resuscitation, defined here as a procedure which restores to life those who have been professionally regarded as dead or as likely to die within minutes were positive steps not taken to intervene artificially to maintain respiration and circulation. It too, like euthanasia, has to be undertaken by others, and with or without the consent of the dying person. Carrying it out involves the exercise of decision-making by those who, on the basis of consensual, but usually only tacit, agreement have been entrusted with the power and authority to take such decisions. Those so endowed are likely to be guided by implicit or explicit share value-judgments on the quality – the worthiness – of the present and probable future of the lives which are prolonged. Like euthanasia, and for much the same kinds of reason, resuscitation is much more likely to be perceived as a problematic issue in the case of older than of younger people. In general, the quality and hence value of the lives to be saved are likely to be more negatively judged the older the individual concerned.

The issues I want to consider in more detail, however, centre on the question of how far it is morally justified to use *chronological age*, *per se*, as the prime criterion in determining what kind of medical service should be available to individuals, and who should deliver it. They are threefold and interconnected. In discussing them, I will draw *inter alia* on the experiences and opinions that were expressed either in the interviews which I and my colleagues conducted with those who played a part in the development of the geriatric medicine specialty, including those who were critical of some aspects of that development, and in the literature which we examined.

The *first* is the moral legitimacy of the age criterion as a method of rationing scarce medical and surgical procedures which are known to be efficacious in the treatment of adults of all ages. The *second* revolves around the provision of age-segregated facilities for general medical and nursing care, the existence of which are often used as an excuse to exclude access to appropriate specialist advice unquestioningly available to the non-segregated person. In other words, is age segregation a practice that results in discrimination against the old? Or is it a necessary device to ensure a fair share of scarce resources to older people?

The *third* concerns broader considerations of generational equity. Does the use of "age" and not only professionally assessed need for medical treatment have different effects depending upon whether the provision and distribution of beneficial health care facilities in national systems can loosely be labelled as either predominantly "command driven" or predominantly "market oriented"? Indeed, does the method a society chooses to use to meet its health care costs and commitments have a bearing on the moral issue of social justice?

Age discrimination in the rationing of scarce treatment facilities

In considering the first issue, the classic case which springs to mind is that of the treatment of patients with end-stage renal failure now that medical advances have made it possible to prolong life and relieve symptoms whether by dialysis or by kidney transplant from a live donor or cadaver. Incidentally, I am here taking for granted that the medical profession and health service personnel generally increasingly accept that their objective is to improve or maintain the *quality* of individuals' lives rather than merely prolong them. This is not *per se* an age issue, although it is more often proclaimed as a specific objective in the care of very old rather than of middle-aged or young patients.

The often-supplied rationale for the mostly implicit decisions which were taken to restrict the procedures to individuals below a certain age usually were that, in general, the older the individual the poorer the likely outcome. The development of QALYs (quality-adjusted life years)[3] by economists as an explicit measure which can be used in determining the relative benefit of undertaking one kind of action rather than another has conveniently given some post-hoc justification to the use of the age criterion as a rationing device. While the use of QALY criteria is not yet universally acceptable, it seems to have provided a way in which chronological age can be included in priority assessments without being morally discriminating. Before the specification of QALY-determined values it had been generally assumed that the survival of the young, whatever the quality of the young lives involved, was more desirable than the amelioration of the lives of older people. Using QALY-type calculations – for example to evaluate the cost utility of hip replacements, required mainly by older people, as against the treatment of accidentally acquired severe brain damage, most of whose victims were young men – has had the effect of legitimising and encouraging the shift of resources into orthopaedic surgery affecting mostly older people. The moral standing of the use of QALY as a method of determining medical priorities, however, is still under close scrutiny. In an examination of the use of a QALY-like standard exercise to determine which Medicaid patients should be able to claim their medical fees from the US State of Oregon suggested that it (the State) would do better to spend money on providing cosmetic breast surgery rather than on repairing fractured femurs.[4]

Let us return to the theme of access to life-enhancing medical measures in the UK. "Age", we were told by our informants in the study we made of geriatric medicine, was used habitually throughout their careers by surgeons and general physicians (and accepted by referring agents like general practitioners) as an overriding blanket criterion to justify excluding older individuals from a variety of clinical procedures which were likely to be just as efficacious among them as among younger people. I understand from talking to someone currently involved in assessing health needs and health gains in the public health directorate of a Thames Regional Health Authority that it remains so. For example, although the health gain from a particular form of efficacious chemotherapeutic treatment following a diagnosis of lung cancer was found to be comparable for 85+ and 65–70-year-olds in one treatment centre, doctors working at the centre selected proportionately twice as many of the latter as of the former for it.

The morality of the age criterion as a determinant of whether or not individuals should be offered treatments of known efficacy is now, however, being more seriously brought into question by recent advances in surgical and medical techniques. For example, it used to be held that older people could not withstand major surgery because their physiological recuperative capacity had deteriorated to such an extent that their lives would be jeopardised were they to be exposed to it. For example, some geriatricians held it to be their role to protect old people from iatrogenically inspired interventions rather than plead support for further interventions on their behalf. Now I am informed by more than one impeccable medical source that advances in anaesthesia and in the use of lasers have reduced the risks which were associated with major surgery and by and large increased with age. It is now possible to submit much older and frailer patients to it than was the case a decade ago. Stances which originally were based on moral grounds – those of not exposing the vulnerable to considerable pain or discomfort if there were only a remote chance of ultimate benefit – are now being re-examined, since the particular circumstances which pertained when they were established have changed.

Age segregation in the hospital sector

The second ethical issue concerns the legitimacy of health service provisions in which those over a certain chronological age presenting with comparable problems to those below that age are treated in different environments and by different medical, nursing and other healing and caring professions from those who have not reached that age. I want to consider whether the creation of facilities specifically designed to provide medical and nursing care for the old, and the creation of a cadre of doctors and nurses whose responsibilities are exclusively the care of the old, can be held to have been a denial of justice to the old or, on the contrary, a device whereby the socio-biological disadvantaging of the old has by such measures been mitigated and reduced.

Both views have been voiced ever since the setting up of the NHS, and are still being voiced by members of the medical profession and others, as well as by those concerned with social and welfare policies relating to the care of older people. The balance of opinion seems to have swung in recent years against the policy of building a strong geriatric specialty where those engaged in it deal exclusively with older people, and towards one of reintegrating the medical care of older people into that of mainstream general medicine and the body system specialties which are not age based. The latter policy implies that those involved in the care of older people will also be dealing with younger adults. (I do not propose to deal here with the development of paediatrics as a specialty and the expanding interpretation of the upper age boundary of its competency by its proponents, which also raises issues of age discrimination but of a rather different kind. Nevertheless, something can be learned from comparing the case for age-band specialisation at both ends of the age scale.)

To understand the controversy and its salience at any given time it is vital to consider the changing historical context in which the arguments have been embedded. To begin with it is necessary to remember what the legacy of medical care provision at the start of the NHS was like in 1948. There were two kinds of hospital provision. By 1939, voluntary hospitals almost exclusively admitted patients requiring acute medical or surgical treatment. Such hospitals sought deliberately to exclude those who were likely to be labelled medically the chronically sick or incurable as well as those with highly infectious diseases. The fate of those labelled "chronic sick", the great majority of whom were the "aged poor", was in the hands of local authority hospitals, most of which until 1929 had been poor law infirmaries. The younger patients in local authority hospitals were mostly to be found in fever hospitals or in those specialising in tuberculosis management. As reported to us in our survey, the general assumption at the time, and one shared by most members of the medical profession whose training had taken place exclusively in the most prestigious voluntary hospitals, was that sickness in old age was synonymous with chronicity and incurability. It therefore merited only what can crudely be considered "warehousing" rather than active treatment. In a nutshell, the pre-1948 legacy, therefore, had resulted in a predominantly segregated service where old, frail individuals could at best expect benign guardianship until they died rather than active treatment aimed at their ultimate discharge.

The first serious challenge to the validity of the customary equation of old age with chronicity occurred during the war years from Drs Marjory Warren and Lionel Cosin. As superintendents of local authority hospitals which had only recently been poor law infirmaries they had medical responsibility for the care of most hospitalised chronic sick patients. In the institutions for which they were responsible they began to show that if elderly people, who had been considered incurable, were given a thorough medical examination and diagnosis and rehabilitative activities, many of them were able to respond positively to steps taken by nurses and paramedical therapists to restore atrophied physical capacities and regain the desire to become more independent by taking up once more the personal hygiene and domestic management tasks required for independent or quasi-independent living in their own homes or in non-medically controlled residential institutions.

These discoveries gave those who pioneered their implementation the confidence to claim that the customary segregationist practice of pre-NHS days, which minimalised the access of older people, particularly of the lower social classes, to active medical interventions was no longer justifiable, at least on *medical* grounds. Its perpetuation could only be explained either, on the one hand, by the persistence of a reluctance on the part of the medical and nursing professions to work with and for older people, or, on the other hand, by the heritage of segregated institutions which successive governments were willing to accept as ethically permissible when health care costs were considered to be rising exponentially and in need of control. There was also, reputedly, a widespread dread of hospitals by older people since their parents had only entered them to die rather than obtain treatment.

The strategy of the first generation of geriatricians was therefore to bring the medical care of elderly people into the orbit of the *general* hospital sector, comprising first and foremost the erstwhile voluntary hospitals, and at the same time to press for more resources and better facilities in those hospitals once controlled by local authorities, which still catered for most of those who were over pensionable age.

To do this they pressed for the appointment of consultants with designated responsibilities for geriatric medicine. Initially there was controversy among them as to whether tactically they would achieve more by advocating the allocation of consultant posts to general physicians with an *interest in geriatric care* or should press for appointments *exclusively in geriatric medicine*. In favour of the first, it could be argued that they were likely to receive more support from general physicians *and* attract a higher proportion of the profession's young "high fliers" into the medical care of old people. In favour of the second, it was argued that, if the decisions as to how much medical resource was to be spent on the treatment of older and younger individuals were to be left to the whims of individual, unregenerated general physicians, in the prevailing climate of attitudes to old age and chronic sickness older people would not get as much of their attention as would younger patients. In their view, old people could only be guaranteed reasonable and fair access to medical resources if there was specific institutional provision for them – provision which should also include specialists in treating old people whose needs and responses might differ from those of younger people with comparable diagnoses.

Papers read at the annual conferences of the Medical Society for the Care of the Elderly from its foundation in 1947 until its translation into the British Geriatric Society in 1959 reflect the controversy, which has continued ever since and has not yet been resolved. At first, the arguments were finely balanced and the Regional Health Authorities varied their practice, some of them initially making appointments of general physicians with a special interest; others gave consultant status in geriatric medicine to those who had been medical superintendents of old poor law infirmaries. The majority of the former were given consultant posts based in district general hospitals that had their origin in the voluntary sector: the majority of the latter were located in hospitals which had always been in the public sector.

In the 1960s and early 1970s, when more money was being made available to the NHS and when support for the main tenets of the post-Second World War Welfare State was still bipartisan, politically speaking, the advocates of undiluted specialism were the more successful. The Welfare State ideology emphasised the responsibility of the State, at national and local level, deliberately to transfer resources to the disadvantaged, including the increasing number of very old people. During those years, there was a greater expansion of geriatric than of general medicine consultant posts in the district general hospitals. Training posts in the form of junior hospital doctor staff complements increased to support the consultant posts. Little by little, parallel moves took place in academia. University medical faculties established departments and chairs in geriatrics, which added to its respectability. Medical students for the first time on any scale were exposed to clinical teaching in geriatric wards. A sub-specialty of psychiatry – psychogeriatrics – began to develop and to be given resources in the form of consultant posts that were held in either the district general or in the ex-local authority hospitals or in both. Moreover, there was little resistance to the disproportional expansion of geriatric posts on the part of general physicians because they were apt to see the older patients who had somehow found their way into their beds as "bed blockers". From this perspective, the development of geriatric wards within the same hospitals indicated an acceptable way of removing them without being accused of the inhuman treatment of older, defenceless people.

Since the 1980s, however, there has once again been something of a shift in the views expressed in and outside the specialty. Some leading academic physicians, including those whose primary reputation has been based on their substantial contribution to the theory and practice of geriatric medicine, have argued – and their arguments have been given considerable attention by the influential Royal College of Physicians of London – that the separation of geriatric medicine from general medicine no longer best serves the interests of old people, if it ever did.

Their reasoning is partly based on their belief that recent developments in medicine and surgery are such that older people could benefit from them and could be more likely to do so if they were to be admitted to beds under the supervision of general or body-system medical and surgical specialists rather than to geriatric wards which are still frequently in parts of hospital settings some distance from the high-tech diagnostic and treatment facilities.

They also argue that the experience of the last twenty years indicates that the prospect of exclusive responsibility for the care and treatment of older people, despite the efforts of geriatricians to enthuse neophytes, still does not attract sufficient numbers of the most enterprising young medical graduates, with the result that older people admitted to geriatric wards can be denied the expertise of the most forward-looking doctors.

The argument is also made that there is an inevitable arbitrariness in the decisions which *de facto* have to be made as to which patients are appropriately admitted to geriatric wards and which to those allocated to general medicine physicians or other specialists. Some district health authorities (DHAs), in seeking to regulate their purchasing activities with provider hospitals, have imposed an arbitrary rule which relegates all those above 75 or 80 years of age to the geriatric wards of the hospitals, whether these are directly under their control or Trust providers with whom they have contracts.

General practitioners in the past have been, and at least those among them who are budget holders in the future will continue to be, important informal arbiters as to where old people are referred, because they enjoy the freedom to make contracts with hospitals and to refer to particular consultants' outpatient clinics. There is likely to be strong pressure on "budget holding" general practitioners, however, from the DHAs and the hospitals themselves to conform to official guidelines concerning chronological age, irrespective of their own opinions on the specific needs of their individual patients. And, as everyone agrees, some 80-year-olds have a physical and mental status more like that of the average 65-year-old, while others more closely resemble a typical 90-year-old.

There are still other arguments which suggest that the separate status of geriatric medicine is no longer appropriate and fair from a natural justice point of view, even if it once was. For example, evidence is accumulating to suggest that the survivors into their 80s today are in general healthier than those of a generation ago, but that those who are acutely ill are likely either to require short-term, intensive medical and nursing care in a terminal illness of the kind now available unquestioningly to younger people, or social support best delivered to them either in their own homes or in residential care homes which are now more abundant than they once were. Consequently, so the argument goes, the need to concentrate on the restoration of functional capacity by staff employed in the hospital sector, where stays are essentially short term, is no longer as salient as it once was.

These arguments are undoubtedly carrying increasing weight with health authorities responsible for assessing need and planning how to meet their obligations to provide effective services to the population, which is already an ageing population and likely to remain so in the future. By "an ageing population" is meant that the proportion of very old people (those over 80) has increased substantially in the last decades and is expected to increase still further in the next few. It should be remembered, however, that the way in which the population ageing process is occurring is often presented by professional people as well as by politicians and the media in such a way as to produce unnecessary panic about its economic and social costs. In numerical terms, a two-thirds increase between 1985 and 2001 in the numbers of 85-year-olds and older in the population of Great Britain means that 17 in every 1000 of the total population will be in that age bracket in year 2001, compared with 11 in 1985. Viewed in this way, it is permissible to ask whether a country as technologically advanced and competent as ours cannot encompass that increase without demanding undue sacrifices from the rest of the community. In the last analysis it depends upon the relative values attached to securing a dignified and tranquil life for those who survive to a great age.

There are, however, cogent arguments on the other side, that is, from those who believe that the development of a specialty was an essential step in ending the pre-NHS *de facto* exclusion of most old people from appropriate forms of medical and nursing care. They believe that its separate status is still essential if advances in medical knowledge and skills of direct benefit to the very elderly are to be sustained. The argument is that if physicians had had patients of all ages exclusively under their care during the whole of the post-war period, given prevailing social values, they would not have given sufficient attention to the problems which elderly people alone face or face in greater measure than younger people. The proponents of this view claim it was only the exclusive concentration on the problems associated with illness in the elderly which enabled advances now taken for granted to be made. Some also argue that, given contemporary ambivalent attitudes to old age – whether these attitudes are biologically in-built or socially induced is not material to the argument – not all those who enter medicine or nursing, and do valuable work in it, are temperamentally capable of relating to old people at a personal level, and hence would be unable to provide effective services in this field.

They claim, moreover, that the specialty has been particularly successful in ensuring that a fair share of scarce resources is set aside for the medical care of older people, and that they have been more successful than general physicians in what is now called "networking", that is in considering with others both inside and outside the health service proper the multiple socio-medical requirements of older people. To disband it by letting the specialty be reabsorbed into the general body of general medicine specialists could, they argue, jeopardise the advances in inter-sectoral and inter-professional collaboration which have been laboriously established in the past decades, and need to go further.

In short, the arguments both for and against the perpetuation of a medical specialty of geriatrics are nicely balanced. It is difficult to claim moral superiority in the form of greater or lesser degrees of social justice for one or the other as both sides have attempted to do. The dominance of one or other at any given time appears to owe more to issues relating to the perceived self-interests of particular sections of the medical profession and their success in persuading decision-making authorities at national and local level that their proposals are more likely than those of their opponents to obtain tacit popular support as well as serve the interests of elderly people, their relatives and the community at large.

Generational equity and the philosophy of health care provision

I now come to the third and final issue, broadly defined as that of generational equity. The philosophy behind the Welfare State exemplified in the language of the 1948 NHS Act was that health and some other basic services should be available according to individuals' intrinsic needs for them and not according to the demand for them which individuals could express by the utilisation of their own purchasing power.

Given that these worthy objectives have not been achieved in full across all age bands, does this mean that the system for providing health care for the population at large installed in the UK in the post-war period has achieved less generational equity in the distribution of health care resources than have other national systems for funding and providing health care?

It is worth noting that in the United States, where the health services are more "market oriented", and not "command driven" as they are in the UK, much less stress has been placed on age as a criterion for determining whether or not treatment is given to or withheld from patients with end-stage renal failure. There the capacity of the individual to pay appears in practice to have been a much more relevant consideration whether to institute treatment, especially on a long-term basis, as in dialysis, than it would have been in the UK. But lobby pressure on behalf of some disadvantaged groups has also induced the US federal government to introduce some programmes for those with chronic illnesses, which are more generously funded that their equivalents in Britain. Although the cult of youth appears in many ways to be even stronger in the United States that it does in Britain, more regard seems to have been paid in the former country to the dignity of old age. For example, perhaps due to the lobbying activities of the grey panthers, there has been a greater diminution in the use of chronological age to exclude individuals wishing to participate in the satisfying domains of work and leisure.

And has the development within our health care system of an institutionalised medical specialty to deal with the care of older people helped to reduce the inequalities in their access to the best quality of medicine that can be produced, an inequality which undoubted existed at the outset of the NHS, to a greater or lesser extent than the inequalities which also existed and continue to exist elsewhere in the developed world? Or has the British development, seen primarily as benign by some overseas observers[5] as well as by the native, possibly biased geriatric lobby, meant that older people have failed to get a fair share of the improvements which have taken place over the years in the capacity of medicine to meet the medical needs of the population?

Notes and references

1. The study has been financially supported by a generous grant from the Wellcome Trust.
2. The controversy concerning whether or not there is convincing evidence that technologically advanced countries are now nearing the time when a majority of its men and women can expect to reach the human species' natural life span is well rehearsed by Michael Bury in a chapter entitled "Arguments about ageing: long life and its consequences" in N. Wells and C. Freer (eds), *The Ageing Population* (Macmillan, London 1988).
3. The development of QALYs as an outcome measure for judging the cost-effectiveness of medical interventions has been primarily developed by Alan Williams and his economist colleagues at the Centre for Health Economics at the University of York. See Williams, "Economics of coronary artery bypass grafting" (1985) 291 *British Medical Journal* 326–9.
4. The Oregon scheme is well described by Dixon and Welch, "Priority setting: lessons from Oregon" (1991) 337 *Lancet* 891–4.
5. Cf. W. H. Barker, "Adding life to years: organized geriatric services" in *Great Britain and Implications for the United States* (Johns Hopkins Press, Baltimore 1987).

The development and future of research ethics committees in Britain

Claire Gilbert Foster

An author once said of the characters in his novels that they seemed, after he had created them, to take on an independent existence and to determine their own destinies, in a way over which he had little control. The same could be said of the numerous research ethics committees that have proliferated all over Britain since the late 1960s.

The development of ethical review

Early measures

In 1963 Sir Austin Bradford-Hill (Professor Emeritus of Medical Statistics, University of London) gave the Marc Daniels Lecture, entitled "Medical Ethics and Controlled Trials".[1] In it he argued against the implementation of the proposed World Medical Association's Declaration of Helsinki.[2] He said that no code could anticipate and deal with every situation that arose in medical research, and any code would unnecessarily limit and constrain research for that reason. One of the points he picked upon on the proposed Declaration was informed consent. He said:[3]

> Personally, and speaking as a patient, I have no doubt whatever that there are circumstances in which the patient's consent to

Choices and Decisions in Health Care. Edited by A. Grubb.

> taking part in a controlled trial should be sought. I have equally no doubt that there are circumstances in which it need not – and even should not – be sought ... Surely it is often quite impossible to tell ill-educated and sick persons the pros and cons of a new and unknown treatment versus the orthodox and known? And in fact, of course one does not know ... Can you describe that situation to a patient so that he does not lose confidence in you – the essence of the doctor/patient relationship – and in such a way that he fully understands and can therefore give an *understanding* consent to his inclusion in the trial? In my opinion nothing less is of value. Just to ask the patient does he mind if you try some new tablets on him does nothing, I suggest, to meet the problem ... If the patient cannot really grasp the whole situation, or without upsetting his faith in your judgment cannot be made to grasp it, then in my opinion the ethical decision still lies with the doctor, whether or not it is proper to exhibit, or withhold a treatment.

Sir Austin Bradford-Hill went on to say that a code telling doctors that they must always obtain informed consent takes no heed of the "enormously varying circumstances of clinical medicine".[4]

Three months later, in an editorial, the *British Medical Journal* retorted:[5]

> By his remarks about *not* telling patients of the whys and wherefores of an experiment, Sir Austin has attracted the attention of Mrs. Helen Hodgson, chairman of the Patients' Association, who in the *British Medical Journal* of May 18 sharply challenged him. Mrs Hodgson, according to article in *The Times* (June 17) headed "Now a Voice for the Patient", is moving forward with some determination. A questionary is being sent out to members of the Patients' Association which says this: "Clinical trials are obviously going on, and on a big scale. Patients are not told if they are receiving new or orthodox treatment. I maintain that they should be told. I think it begs the question to say that it is difficult to explain these things to ignorant and sick people." We agree with Mrs Hodgson.

Meanwhile the Royal College of Physicians issued a Report[7] to boards of governors, medical school councils, hospital management committees or equivalent bodies in non-medical institutions, quoted the Surgeon General of the United States who in 1966 had called upon the institutions which funded research to take full ethical responsibility for that research. The Report said that medical institutions had a responsibility for ensuring that all clinical investigations carried out within their hospitals were ethical and conducted with the optimum technical skill and precautions for safety. The report then states:[8]

> This responsibility would be discharged if in medical institutions where clinical investigation is carried out, it were ensured that all projects were approved by a group of doctors including those experienced in clinical investigation. This group should satisfy itself of the ethics of all proposed investigations.

This report was issued in 1967. The Ministry of Health took up the interest of the Royal College of Physicians in creating review bodies, and the following year sent a health notice to regional and area health authorities and to boards of governors asking them to set up research ethics committees.[9] Neither the Royal College of Physicians nor the Ministry of Health, at this stage, would give clear guidance on how these review bodies should work. The Royal College of Physicians' report referred clinical investigators to a statement published in 1964 by the Medical Research Council[10] about ethical research, and to the Declaration of Helsinki.[11] The report added: "However, because of the wide varieties of research, formal codes can only provide general guidance, and their application to specific problems must often remain a matter of opinion."[12] The Ministry of Health circular referred its readers to the Royal College of Physicians' report for more detail.[13]

In 1975 when the Ministry of Health sent a reminder to health districts of the need for independent review, a slightly more detailed set of guidelines on the composition of committees, written by a working party of the Royal College of Physicians, was included.[14] This asked that a lay member (defined as "an individual who is not associated with the profession in any paramedical activity") be included.[15] It also gave some guidance on consent procedures, thereby establishing the importance of obtaining consent from patients, but there was still no guidance about the way committees should run.

The role of research ethics committees was therefore initially defined, by implication, to meet two negative needs – the need not to compromise standards of practice in quest of novel therapies, and the need not to regard the patient "merely as a means" to a desirable end.[16] For Kant, it is permissible to use someone as a means to an end, but only if he shares your end or consents to it. Otherwise, without consent, you are using him "merely as a means".[17] Thus the early emphasis on consent provided research ethics committees with a foundation for a deontological, rather than utilitarian, approach to ethical issues, which some of them have taken further, as we shall see. This did not, however, provide a formula for the good practice of research ethics committees. They were left to work out their own methods. The degree of examination of research proposals would depend on what they considered to be acceptable behaviour by researchers and to what extent they could be trusted to behave well without being told. Committees would make their own decisions about their own standing orders. They would decide if and how often they should meet, what questions they should ask about the research proposal, whether they should just look together at each research protocol or whether they needed to interview the researcher as well. Some committees devised an application form for the researcher to complete so as to ensure that all the issues they believed to be important were covered. All these details would have been decided on the basis of what each committee perceived its role to be, and, needless to say, each committee could have had a slightly different view of this. Diversity of practice was therefore inherent in the system of ethical review right from the beginning.

In the United States, it was the same statement by the Surgeon-General in 1966[18] that had inspired the creation of peer review committees (called institutional review boards). Unlike Britain, however, the move to create these boards was very much more centrally organised and engineered. By 1974 a new Part 46 was added to Subtitle A of Title 45 of the Code of Federal Regulations, stating that no Department of Health, Education and Welfare funded grant or contract involving subjects at risk could be undertaken unless a committee at the institution reviewed the proposal. Details about what the review should consist of were also made clear in Part 46. Concern that the committees, having been given this power, should make correct decisions about the research they reviewed, was reflected in the creation, two months after Part 46 was written, of the National Commission for the Protection of Human Subjects of Biomedical and Behavioural Research. This commission became active in assessing and amending federal regulations on the protection of human subjects. Thus the May 1974 rules contained 22 sections, whereas the most recent rules of January 1981 contain 38 sections.[19]

We can see, then, that the approach to ethical review of research in the United States was quite opposite to that taken by Britain. In the United States the notion was enshrined in law from the beginning, and the rules governing it were amended as experience grew. In Britain an attitude of "wait and see" was prevalent, so that research ethics committees have had to develop their own rules as they went along. It is only in 1992 that the British government, through the Department of Health, has put any concerted effort into making policy decisions on behalf of research ethics committees.[20]

Royal College of Physicians' guidelines 1984 and 1990

By 1984, when the first really detailed guidelines were issued by the Royal College of Physicians,[21] many research ethics committees had been working for some time, and had developed and refined their methods through experience and practice.

The 1984 guidelines of the college made a number of points clear: (1) by which ethical principles committees were to abide; (2) that they were to look at, *inter alia*, the scientific quality of the research; (3) that they must look at *all* research projects in their districts; (4) the definition of a research project; (5) who should be members of the committees; (6) who should nominate the members; (7) what questions the committees should ask of the research; (8) how the committees should work, including the need to meet regularly, to keep accurate records of the meetings and a host of other standing orders; (9) how to deal with research on vulnerable groups; (10) the need for informed consent, and a number of miscellaneous topics in addition. But by this time many research ethics committees had developed their own idiosyncrasies and were fiercely independent. The guidelines were not binding and were not automatically followed, so they did not draw research ethics committees into line with each other. Surveys during the 1980s indicated that knowledge of the Royal College of Physicians' guidelines was not universal and that many research ethics committees were simply ignoring the guidance they contained.[22] Julia Neuberger's 1990–1991 survey[23] shows a similar pattern of idiosyncratic behaviour. By the time she did her survey, the Royal College of Physicians had issued three more sets of guidelines: an updated version of their 1984 publication,[24] guidance for research on healthy volunteers[25] and for research on patients.[26] The Association of British Pharmaceutical Industries had also published a series of guidelines,[27] as had the British Medical Association[28] and the General Medical Council.[29]

Department of Health circular 1991

Fierce independence continues to be a hallmark of research ethics committees in Britain. Early responses to more comprehensive guidelines finally issued in 1991 by the Department of Health[30] and circulated to all district health management committees indicate that research ethics committees respect the weight the guidelines carry, but that they are not intending to follow them to the letter. As with other guidelines, research ethics committees are discriminating about which parts of the guidelines they will follow and which they will circumvent. Many committees, for example, are not meeting the request made in the department's guidelines to make either the chairman or the vice-chairman a lay person. There several reasons given for this: one is that committees do not feel that the lay person can adequately fulfil the role of chairman because of his necessary lack of medical knowledge; another is that the lay person can be more effective in discussions if he or she does not have the chair, since the lay person's contribution often consists of asking difficult questions; another is that to have either the chairman's or vice-chairman's post always filled by one of two or three members of the committee is limiting and undemocratic. Other reasons are given but the important point to note is that committees do not automatically follow guidelines even when they come from the government.

Weaknesses in the British system of ethical review

There has been a proliferation of research ethics committees within and outside the National Health Service with no central registering mechanism or legal framework, and therefore nothing, save poorly implemented guidelines, to bring committees into line with each other. There is concern that research ethics committees are not all functioning adequately, but there is no way of knowing which are not, and there is no agreed method by which to ensure that they do so. Equally, there are no means by which to accredit research ethics committees that are working well. Moreover, these better, usually longer established, committees have gained a wealth of experience in the methodical scrutiny of the ethics of a wide variety of research projects, but have no opportunity to share that experience with newer committees. There should be no need for every committee to go through the lengthy process of discovery and refinement of the early committees, but currently there are no means by which committees can build on the experience of each other.

This isolation of research ethics committees has the result that, most of them being well intentioned and hard working, each tends to believe that its own methods are all right. Some committees still do not hold meetings, but leave their chairmen to decide which protocols need scrutiny by other members of the committee and which do not, only sending those that do to members for comments. These committees will argue that no unethical research has been approved by this method. In isolation the argument that this is a perfectly valid way of working may be won, at least with the individual members' consciences, if not with published guidelines. The chairmen will, in most cases, know when the procedures of the research will be harmful. No research would be approved which actually harmed its subjects. But is this sufficient? Many committees would now argue that it is not.

An exact definition of an effective research ethics committee does not exist. Nobody has defined exactly what constitutes an effective research ethics committee; how it can ensure that research is ethical; which issues it must cover when reviewing projects; what the solutions are in every case. It has been only by means of trial and error, reflection and an openness to redefining viewpoints that research ethics committees have continued to develop and improve. Twenty years ago a committee which did not meet, whose members only swiftly perused a research protocol to ensure that no physical damage was likely to be done to the research subjects, may have been perfectly acceptable. Now it is not thought that merely ensuring that nothing harmful will be done to research subjects is sufficient. There has been an unmistakable shift from a utilitarian approach, in which it is acceptable to subsume the individual needs of a few patients to the good of many future patients, provided they are protected from harm and the end is socially desirable. Committees are becoming more Kantian, in that they are beginning to acknowledge that any use of people "merely as a means"[31] is unacceptable. This view would conclude, in its purest form, that even the most non-invasive research, which it is unlikely that a subject would refuse, should not be approved by the committee, *unless* the subjects are to be made aware of what it proposed, and give their explicit consent to it. In Kantian terms: they would then be being used as a means without being used "merely as a means",[32] and the strong Kantian requirement that subjects should share the end of the researchers is fulfilled. This is not yet an established view among committees but attitudes are moving towards it. Many committees are beginning to interpret their role as protectors of the subject population more radically: aiming to protect their autonomy as well as their welfare. There is a growing recognition of the moral distinction between the idea of *harming* a person (either in the purely physical sense or by damaging his interests) and that of *wronging* him (by infringing his autonomy).

In the next section I will show how research ethics committees have begun to meet resistance from researchers who maintain the utilitarian view which the committees are beginning to question. At this point I would emphasise that this shift is taking place only in some committees and they are left to themselves to work out the implications of the shift. The diversity between committees is therefore increasing as the more reflective committees change their practices in accordance with their views, and the other committees are doubly disadvantaged. First, by their unprofessional methods they are already working at a level unacceptable to most persons involved in, or subject to, research. Secondly, because they do not have the opportunity to reconsider and discuss issues as they arise in meetings they are far less likely to change their approaches and methods. No external structure exists which will reach out to these committees and teach them to change.

The diversity and independence of research ethics committees has led to a series of difficulties faced by those organising large-scale research. The following is an extract from a report on an omni-centre study (where the research is organised from one place and carried out by one person or a group of persons in one place all over the country) of the national risk factor of listeriosis:

> The study was to be non-invasive, simply involving interviews with cases and suitably matched controls. The questions were mainly about food intake and were not intrusive or sensitive; however, because the subjects had recently undergone a major life event, ethical approval was sought ...

The protocol, which had been written in late 1988, was submitted to the next available meeting of the Public Health Laboratory Service (PHLS) ethics committee in early 1989. Approval was not granted: the committee asked for a re-submission in which the protocol was to be amended to indicate that it would be submitted to local ethics committees. The principal researcher asked for this view to be reconsidered since it would necessitate contacting some 200 bodies, some of which met infrequently and all of which had different procedures, thereby placing impossible constraints upon an urgently required study.

This point was accepted and it was proposed that the case could be met by placing a notice about the study in the [in-house] journal. This was done at the end of December 1989; the notice outlined the purpose and methodology and invited readers to ask [the researcher] to provide a formal local ethics committee submission if they felt it necessary.

In the event, 46 districts responded: 4 indicated that they were happy for the study to be undertaken without requiring further details, 25 simply requested the study protocol and 17 sent their own ethics committee forms to be completed.

Initial response times to the PHLS notice [in the Report] ranged from 1 to 12 weeks (median 3 weeks), excluding 1 district which asked for a sight of the protocol 42 weeks later. Of the 46 responding districts, 13 had to be prompted to reply after they had been sent the protocol or completed forms, entailing a great deal of telephone time attempting to contact chairpersons. In order to reach one, six 'phone calls were made, as initially no-one appeared to either know him or where he could be contacted. Such difficulties were particularly prevalent where (as in this case) the chairperson was non-medical.

The 17 districts who had sent forms all replied within 12 weeks of despatch of the completed form, but those who had requested the protocol had a median response time of 15 weeks (range 3 weeks–11 months).

Channels of communication frequently became blocked; 1 district lost our paperwork, another committee's secretary had filed the papers away so the study was not discussed at the next appropriate meeting. Seven committees approved the study, but failed to inform us until prompted, including one where, although the study had been approved within 3 weeks of receipt of the protocol, we were not informed until almost 4 months later. A similar delay of 3 months occurred with another district.

> There were several idiosyncrasies: two committees required a principal investigator to hold contracts with their Health Authorities; three required minor amendments to the protocol; one required the signature of all consultants whose patients would be involved in the research (impossible to predict in this study); some insisted on written consent forms although the initial national ethics committee had specifically recommended that verbal informed consent was appropriate. One committee, having granted approval, required completion of a further form for the Unit General Manager. Two districts asked for personal attendance of an investigator at the ethics committee meeting (both waived this requirement following telephone conversations with the principal investigator); although each of the 17 formal applications was accompanied by a letter to the chairman stressing the non-invasive nature of the study and its approval by the national committee, in only 5 cases was chairman's action taken.
>
> Two of the 17 "formal application" districts requested 12 (and 2 districts required 10) copies of all the documentation ... Additional costs included telephone calls, photocopying, clerical and medical staff time which was increased by the fact that no two of the 17 ethics committees' forms were the same. Their layout varied greatly – particularly with regard to space provided for answers to essentially similar questions. Furthermore, although there was a basic "core" of approximately 16 questions, their different phrasing meant that, in practice, a total of over 75 had to be answered.
>
> Despite prompting by telephone and letter, one district has yet to respond; another two, when telephoned, "thought" our application was successful, would check to let us know, but nothing more has been heard. We were granted approval by the hospital ethics committee in one district, but are still awaiting a response from the GP ethics committee in the same district.
>
> The study was refused approval by 1 ethics committee in a district which possessed two – the other approved the study! We received no formal letter from the Chairman of the former.

An example of the difficulties of those organising multi-centre research (where the research is carried out in many centres with responsible researchers in each) comes from the Royal College of General Practitioners' Manchester Research Unit. The Royal College of General Practitioners has, unusually, its own Clinical Research Ethics Committee, which looks at GP research proposals which involve more than three centres. It will ordinarily give its approval, if the research is up to standard, and it then informs the local committees in the centres where the research is to take place. In this instance, the research was a form of post-marketing surveillance of a particular use of a licensed drug, and so the local committees were not informed, since they do not have to consider this kind of research, according to the Department of Health guidelines.[33] The following account was given by one of the researchers at the unit:[34]

> We have had a lot of problems with ethical committees, particularly with our latest project, the RCGP Myocardial Infarction Study, which is looking at the use of a thrombolytic (clot-buster) when used to treat patients who have just had a heart attack. The study is primarily a post-marketing surveillance study. Since this study would involve over 4000 general practitioners throughout the United Kingdom, we applied for ethical approval to the RCGP Clinical Research Ethics Committee. Approval was obtained. Since the project has been launched, we have had many letters from chairmen of local ethical committees intimating that we have acted unethically by not approaching them directly. This has caused quite a lot of friction, and in one case has resulted in the chairman of one local ethical committee circularising all general practitioners within his area intimating that our study had not obtained ethical approval. Clearly, these chairmen have not read the Department of Health Guidelines on local ethical committees, which states specifically that company-sponsored post-marketing surveillance studies are exempt from the requirement for local ethical approval.

The level of diversity of research ethics committees, and the lack of agreement and coordination between them, is unacceptable. The problems experienced by clinicians doing multi- or omni-centre research highlight a whole series of faults in the system of ethical review in this country. Indeed, these problems in obtaining ethical approval for large-scale research projects are the best evidence we have so far for the unsatisfactory state of the functioning of research ethics committees.

There are, however, a number of positive aspects to the way research ethics committees have evolved in the UK, which should not be overlooked. Any solution should build on their strengths as well as taking into account their weaknesses and the problems arising therefrom.

Strengths in the British system of ethical review

In avoiding too hasty a definition of how research ethics committees should work in the late 1960s, we have also avoided limiting their scope before we really had any idea of the extent of that scope. We have left committees free to develop as they saw fit, and as a result have numerous examples of strong, independent committees capable of assessing research and engaging in serious ethical discussion. They are also open to considering new developments, and a dynamic method of practice, reflection on practice, and continuing improvement of practice, has ensued. Thus, for example, the shift from protecting the subjects of research just from harm to protecting them from being wronged as well has been reflected in many, though not all, committees.

Research ethics committees are in the vanguard of these changing attitudes. Because they have had to consider what is and what is not ethical in medical research, they have brought into the open many issues relevant to medical ethics. Because most grant-giving bodies and most journals now require researchers to obtain ethical approval prior to funding or publishing their research, the standards set by research ethics committees have to be met. A furious row has been sparked off in some quarters by the fact that research ethics committees demand a far higher level of communication between doctor and patient than the level believed to be normal to clinical practice. This has been seen by some researchers as setting a double standard. They argue that the clinical researcher is more intellectually honest and doing more lasting good than the clinician who does not do research and does not trouble himself about discovering new therapies or re-examining old ones. The researcher goes to the trouble of setting up a controlled trial when he knows there is something to be discovered about the medicine he practises and thereby provides valid scientific evidence which will improve future medical care. Yet he is penalised for his trouble by having to engage in the time-consuming procedure of obtaining informed consent from his recruits. The practitioner who does not do the research has no similar obligation to obtain informed consent – that is, he does have such an obligation but there is no ethics committee insisting upon it and checking on how he will obtain it. The result is that it is much harder to do research than it is not to do research. Not only this, argue the researchers, but further, the practitioner, not informing his patient, is more likely to keep the trust of his patients to whom he presents no doubtful prognoses than the researcher who is obliged to admit uncertainty to his patients. I do not propose to take issue with the various questionable points in these arguments here. What is important to note is that the beliefs of these researchers, that informed consent is not always necessary, only recently went out of date in the medical profession generally, yet research ethics committees are emphatically defending the vital role of informed consent. Thus, in spite of the fury of the debate, the likely outcome will be higher standards of communication in clinical practice rather than lower standards of communication in research. Research ethics committees are not bowing to the pressure of a few researchers who wish to see a lower standard of communication in research, just because it slows down their work. By their insistence that researchers give full and clear information to their potential consenting participants, committees have unquestionably contributed to the education of doctors' attitudes towards the treatment of their patients.

The fierce independence of committees may have made it difficult for guidelines to be accepted, but it has meant that the principle of independent review has been maintained. Most research ethics committees would not dream of surrendering to peer pressure, even when, as in some cases, committees receive a considerable amount of invective because of decisions they have made. They tend not to balk at disapproving or referring back to researchers their unsatisfactory research proposals.

The fact that committees have been left to work out their own methods has meant that members tend to have great loyalty and enthusiasm for their committees, coupled with, generally, a lively defence of their methods.

Proposals for improving the system of ethical review

The need to improve the current system is paramount, for the following reasons. First, it is unacceptable that there should be some research ethics committees which still do not meet adequate standards of practice and therefore expose the general population of potential research subjects to research which is less ethical in the districts for which they are responsible. Secondly, the diversity of committees is a serious check on large-scale research. Thirdly, there now exists a set of guidelines from the European

Commission on good clinical practice in research[35] which will in the future take on the status of a Directive and will, therefore, have to be enacted into law in the UK. These guidelines state on which points researchers must seek an independent committee's opinion. They do not give guidance on methods of working of these committees but the stipulations they make already presuppose a fairly well-structured method. The less adequate committees functioning in the UK will therefore have some trouble in fulfilling the European guidelines when it becomes mandatory to do so.

There is some urgency, then, in providing a solution to the current problems of diversity and inadequacy. There is also a good case for building on the strengths of committees and facilitating their continuing development. The committees themselves, as we have discussed, will not take kindly to external direction. This means that any proposal must meet with the consent and cooperation of research ethics committees themselves. There is, of course, a tension between what those who use research ethics committees perceive to be the needs of committees and what the committees themselves perceive to be their needs. For example, the organisers of large-scale research projects see a real problem in the numerous differences between committees. The committees often hold on to these differences as indicative of their strength. A committee which turns down a proposal for multi-centre research in its district, knowing full well that other committees in other districts have approved the study, is by this very action demonstrating, in its own mind, that it is both more ethical than the other committees and is capable of holding out against the opinions of others when it believes itself to be right. It is also a sign that the committee does its job very thoroughly. That this can be demonstrated is valuable because it means that local researchers will be encouraged to be more careful with their applications in the light of this reputation. Moreover, the committee would be willing and able to defend its decisions, which it may need to do at any time to its appointing authority, to the public, or even before the courts. The self-dependence in the face of contrasting opinions demonstrates how valid is the role of the committee as an independent appraiser. The multi-centre researcher, meanwhile, is stuck with the enormous task of trying to obtain approval for the same protocol from a large number of different research ethics committees.

Those who would improve the functioning of research ethics committees need to remember that the original purpose of these committees was to provide independent review. While more uniformity is unquestionably desirable, the principle of independence should not be lost in the attempt to streamline committees. Moreover, since members of committees may conceivably be personally liable should a case come to court, their own confidence in the decisions they have made and the ways they have come to them is paramount.[36]

I would propose that any attempt to solve the current difficulties with research ethics committees has to meet the following requirements, if it is to succeed:

1. It has to respect the autonomy of committees, and not to work against their independent status.
2. It cannot assume that committees will take notice of directions from outside, unless they see good reasons for so doing.
3. It needs to allow for a dynamic environment in which the issues considered by committees may be continually reassessed in the light of experience and relevant expertise.
4. It should not let the wide experience and sophisticated methods of the more experienced committees go to waste: there is no need to be continually re-inventing the wheel!

The approach should be one of speeding up and facilitating a process that has been taking place for the last thirty years, over a wider area and in a more structured and systematic way.

A minimum standard of practice

The first requirement of any attempt to improve research ethics committees would be to establish and maintain a minimum standard of practice.[37] There needs to be confidence that any committee calling itself a research ethics committee will meet a certain level of practice. At the moment there is nothing to stop any two people calling themselves a research ethics committee and contracting out its services. If a minimum standard could be agreed there would at least be a foundation upon which to build. This standard would need to set the type of people who should be represented on the committee, require that the committee meet regularly, that a consistent method of scrutinising protocols be adopted, that the committee make an annual report available to its appointing authority and to the public, that it has an agreed quorum, that it has accurate minutes of its meetings and that all these matters are enshrined in a written constitution which is available for public scrutiny.

When the European Committee for Proprietary Medicinal Products Guidelines[38] take on the force of a Directive, which they will do at some point, research ethics committees will be obliged to tailor their practices in order to meet the guidelines' requirements within three years. The guidelines do not state approved methods of working. However, their stipulations provide a basis upon which a streamlined application form could be produced. The introduction to the chapter entitled "Protection of Trial Subjects and Consultation of Ethics Committees" states:[39]

> 1.1 The current revision of the Declaration of Helsinki is the accepted basis for clinical trial ethics which must be fully known and followed by all engaged in research on human beings.
>
> 1.2 The personal integrity and welfare of the trial subjects is the ultimate responsibility of the investigator in relation to the trial; but independent assurance that subjects are protected is provided by an ethics committee and freely obtained informed consent.

The guidelines then go on to state that the investigator must request the opinion of relevant ethics committees regarding:

1. suitability of clinical trial products;
2. methods and material used to obtain informed consent from subjects;
3. subsequent protocol amendments and adverse events: whether these would entail additional ethical review;
4. suitability of the investigator, supporting staff and facilities;
5. scientific efficiency of the protocol;
6. justification of risks weighed against benefits to subjects and/or others;
7. how recruitment is to be conducted;
8. how compensation to subjects, insurance and indemnity to cover the investigator will be provided;
9. what reward or compensation investigators and subjects may be offered.

In this chapter there is further clarification of what is meant by informed consent and what is a suitable method for obtaining it.

These very clear guidelines provide the basis for a comprehensive application form for researchers to complete. They do not, note, indicate which are the correct answers to the questions they stipulate research ethics committees should consider, but indicate only upon which points the committees should themselves be satisfied. The independent, responsible status of committees is thereby respected. Should a streamlined form be created prior to the impending Directive, it would make sense to model it upon these guidelines rather than any others.

Given the level of diversity, and the independence of committees, how is the minimum standard even without a streamlined application form to be achieved? It will only work if the committee members themselves have considerable say in the matter. Certainly any attempt, except by means of legislation, to impose standards upon them may be no more (or less) successful than have been existing guidelines. Legislation is likely at some point from Europe[40] but this will take a number of years and meanwhile the British government will almost certainly not legislate before the impending European Directive is issued.

Self-regulation, therefore, is the only really effective option at present. A recognised step towards greater professionalism in other areas has been the creation of an association. There is every reason to suppose that, if committees could be persuaded of its value, a voluntary association of research ethics committees in the UK could be created. Membership would be voluntary, but would be conditional upon a commitment to meet a minimum standard of practice. Therefore, if a committee was a member of the association it would be known that that committee met or was aiming to meet an agreed standard of practice, and this would begin to solve the problem of not knowing how good a committee really is. The association would need to have an executive committee that comprised representatives of members of research ethics committees and to hold an annual general meeting to ratify or rescind decisions of the executive committee. Thereby, any standards would be set by research ethics committee members themselves through the executive committee of the association. Given the level of competence of many committees, these standards would almost certainly be high. Again, this would begin to solve the problem of inadequacy, the degree of diversity would lessen and the desire of committees to regulate their own practices would be fulfilled.

The only obstacle to this approach may be the independence of committees from each other. If they were unwilling to work together in this way, the association could not function. Until an association is formally proposed to the committees themselves their response will not be known. In preliminary interviews with six chairmen of research ethics committees, interest in the idea of an association was shown during conversation with all but one chairman. The reason the one chairman remained doubtful was that her committee members, she felt, would not see how such an association could be of any use to them, since they worked perfectly well already and did not need help from a central body. This is isolationism, not independence, and in the end will not help a committee which professes it. But the more committees that join an association, the more pressure there will be on other committees to join.

Willingness to refine and improve practice

No minimum standard is going to be exactly right, nor indeed will it be sufficient if committees are to continue to provide an adequate service. Many of the more established committees are in the habit of updating their constitutions and application forms regularly, each time rethinking the scope of their role, the questions they really need to ask, and the best ways to phrase these questions. They have demonstrated an openness to change which is invaluable in the work they do, since a concrete definition of their work cannot be found.

Julia Neuberger's survey,[41] and conferences for members of research ethics committees over the last two years, have indicated a general agreement that training should take place. But training is very difficult to devise, given the huge discrepancy in different committees' needs. Some committees would appreciate fairly sophisticated discussions about the difficult cases they have faced; for these committees, basic standing orders have been long established. Other committees need far more rudimentary training on how to run a committee, and there are numerous committees somewhere between these two extremes. With a minimum standard established, however, training could be devised to build from that point and be on offer to committees to take up as they saw fit. A menu of courses could be available, ranging from seminars on different philosophical aspects of ethical review to practical guidance on standing orders.

The process of practice, reflection on practice and improvement of practice could be made universal and speeded up by means of an association. If the association facilitated the free and frequent communication between committees by means of, for example, a newsletter, experiences could be shared and problems solved, not just for one committee, but for all committees which received the newsletter and faced the same problems. Those committees less willing or less interested in self-improvement would be sensitised to the issues they may have thought were outside their remit.

Flexible response to developments

Finally, an association ought to provide a forum within which new developments in medical research, their implications for the work of research ethics committees and the public responses to it can be discussed. All member committees would be kept informed of such developments by means of the newsletter, and responses to them encouraged. The level of experience amongst committees should provide lively and intelligent debate. Committees can themselves indicate areas of need where more information could be made available.

The absence of a central mechanism to look after the needs of research ethics committees is to be strongly deprecated. It is ludicrous that these committees have for so long had no external help whatsoever in their work save for the occasional conference organised by medical ethics centres. An association would be able to facilitate the development of strong and supportive lines of communication between committees, to devise training or literature in response to needs articulated by committees who would have somewhere to turn in order to make their needs known, and would create a forum within which differences and disagreements could be debated in a constructive manner.

Acknowledgement

The author would like to express her gratitude to Sophie Botros for her comments on an earlier draft of this chapter.

Notes and references

1. Bradford-Hill, "Medical ethics and controlled trials" (1963) Marc Daniels Lecture, April 1963.
2. *Declaration of Helsinki: Recommendations Guiding Physicians in Biomedical Research Involving Human Subjects* (World Medical Association, Helsinki, 1964, amended Tokyo, 1975, Venice, 1983 and Hong Kong, 1989).
3. Supra, note 1.
4. Supra, note 1.
5. Editorial, "Ethics of human experimentation" (1963) *British Medical Journal.*
6. Quoted in *Supervision of the Ethics of Clinical Research Investigations in Institutions* (Royal College of Physicians 1967, updated 1973) at p. 5.
7. Ibid.
8. Ibid, at p. 4.
9. HM(68)33, *Supervision of the Ethics of Clinical Trial Investigations* (Ministry of Health, London: HMSO, 1968).
10. *Responsibility in Investigations on Human Subjects* (Report of the Medical Research Council for the year 1962–3, London: HMSO, 1964) at 21–5 (Cmnd 2382).
11. Supra, note 2.
12. Supra, note 6 at p. 3.
13. Supra, note 9 at p. 1.
14. HSC(1S)153 *Supervision of the Ethics of Clinical Research Investigations and Fetal Research* (Department of Health and Social Security, London: HMSO, 1875).
15. Ibid, at p. 3.
16. I. Kant, "*Grounding of the Metaphysic of Morals*", Trans. James W. Ellington Indianapolis: Hackett, 1981.
17. Ibid.
18. Supra, note 6.
19. D. M. Maloney, *Protection of Human Research Subjects* (Plenum Press, New York, 1984) at p. 47.
20. The Department of Health commissioned work in 1992 to review (a) the training needs of members of research ethics committees and (b) policy for assessing the ethics of multi-centre trials. This is the first time that any assessment of the ethical review system in this country has been commissioned by the government.
21. *Guidelines on the Practice of Ethics Committees in Medical Research* (Royal College of Physicians, London, 1984, updated 1990).
22. See R. H. Nicholson (ed.) *Medical Research on Children: Ethics, Law and Practice* (Oxford Medical Publications, Oxford, 1986) and Gilbert, Fulford and Parker, "Diversity in the Practice of District Ethics Committees" (1989) 299 *British Medical Journal* 1437.
23. J. Neuberger, *Ethics Committees in the United Kingdom* (King's Fund, 1992).

24. Supra, note 21.
25. *Research on Healthy Volunteers* (Royal College of Physicians, London, 1986).
26. *Research on Patients* (Royal College of Physicians, London, 1990).
27. Now available in book form: F. O. Wells (ed.), *Medicines: Good Practice Guidelines* (Medical Science Publishing, Belfast, 1990).
28. *Improving the Network of Local Ethical Research Committees and the Establishment of a National Ethical Research Committee* (British Medical Association Central Ethics Committee, London, 1986).
29. *Local Ethics Committees* (General Medical Council, London, 1981).
30. HS6(91)5 *Local Research Ethics Committees* (Department of Health, London, 1991).
31. Supra, note 16.
32. Ibid.
33. Supra, note 30 at p. 19.
34. In correspondence with the author.
35. 111/3976/88-EN, *Guidelines on Good Clinical Practice for Trials on Medicinal Products in the European Community* (European Committee for Proprietary Medicinal Products, implemented 1 July 1991).
36. See, for example, *R* v. *Ethical Committee of St. Mary's Hospital (Manchester), ex p H* [1988] 1 FLR 512 (judicial review of decision to refuse patient access to infertility treatment).
37. See, Kennedy, 'Legal Requirements of Research Ethics Committees' in C. Gilbert Foster (ed.), *Manual for Research Ethics Committees* (King's College, London, 1992).
38. Supra, note 35.
39. Supra, note 35 at p. 13.
40. Supra, note 35.
41. Supra, note 23.

Innovations in procedure and practice in multi-party medical cases

Ken Oliphant

The story begins with Opren. It was the Opren litigation that provided the catalyst for renewed efforts to devise a special set of rules to govern the litigation of multi-party medical cases (MMCs).[1] Opren (short for "Benoxaprofen") was a pharmaceutical manufactured by Eli Lilly & Co. for prescription to those suffering from arthritis. A number of those who took the drug alleged they suffered side-effects, particularly photosensitivity but also liver or kidney failure, leading in some cases to death. The drug was withdrawn from sale in August 1982 and the following year legal proceedings were commenced in the United States. The United States is a favoured forum for tort victims, particularly because trial by jury is the norm.[2] It is thought that juries are more likely than judges to give a "sympathy" verdict to the injured plaintiff in the face of the letter of the law. Furthermore, juries might well be persuaded to award a large sum as exemplary damages designed to punish the defendant rather than merely to compensate the plaintiffs. In England, by contrast, personal injury trials are held in front of a judge sitting without a jury and exemplary damages are regarded as wholly exceptional. It was thus to the chagrin of the English Opren plaintiffs that the American courts refused to grant them forum.

In 1985 proceedings were begun in England instead. MMCs

Choices and Decisions in Health Care. Edited by A. Grubb.

had come before the English courts before (notably in connection with the Thalidomide tragedy)[3] but there was still no special procedure for dealing with the extraordinary problems they posed. The assigned judge, Hirst J, took the innovative step of developing an *ad hoc* procedure, to be known as "the Opren scheme", to make things easier for all concerned. The benefits of this scheme were to be available to those who gave notice of their intention to join by a certain cut-off date. Some 1500 people eventually signed up. Six lead firms of solicitors represented the substantial majority of these, but they also had to liaise with over 200 other solicitors who represented the remaining members of the scheme. On 9 December 1987, Hirst J took the exceptional step of announcing in open court that Eli Lilly had made an offer of an unspecified global sum in full and final settlement of the claims of all those in the scheme and that the six lead firms proposed to recommend acceptance of the offer to their clients and to the other solicitors.[4] The entitlement of each individual plaintiff to damages was to be determined by the six lead firms by reference to the seriousness of the injury as described in the plaintiff's medical report. The basis for assessment was to be the normal measure of tort damages for injuries of the sort suffered, less a "discount for settlement" to take into account the risk the action would have failed had it continued to trial and the benefit of accelerated payment. In case of dispute, the court would act as final arbitrator. A month after making this announcement, the judge welcomed the news that the settlement had been accepted by over 1000 of the plaintiffs, which was a sufficient number to make the settlement effective; he urged the remaining plaintiffs to take advantage of their opportunity to join.[5] This, however, was not the end of the litigation. Since that time, the courts have had to consider the entitlement to legal aid of those who declined to accept the settlement offer, preferring to pursue their claims through the courts instead,[6] and have recognised a "new Opren scheme" for those who started their action too late to join the original scheme.[7]

Undeniably, the Opren litigation has taxed the endurance of the legal system. A LEXIS search suggests that it has necessitated 13 separate hearings in English courts alone. In the course of over six years, the courts considered a mind-boggling variety of issues, amongst them: might the Opren Action Group legitimately take out a full-page advertisement in *The Times* to castigate Eli Lilly for its callous attitude to the litigation?[8]; could the defendants raise objections to the plaintiffs' choice of a particular medical journalist, alleged to have conducted a crusade against the pharmaceutical industry, to sift through the documents supplied by the defendants?[9]; how precisely should the word "Opren" be pronounced?[10] (The answer to this last crucial question, according to Hidden J, was that although a long "O" as in "open" was technically correct it was better to follow common usage and make the "O" short as in "opera".)[11]

This chapter attempts an interim assessment of how successful the English legal system has been in dealing with cases like Opren. Its focus is upon injuries arising out of the use of pharmaceuticals and other medical products; however, many of the issues raised are common to other "mass products cases" (like asbestos) and indeed to some "mass disaster" cases (like the *Herald of Free Enterprise* or King's Cross cases).[12] The scheme of this chapter is as follows: first to identify those features of MMCs that give rise to particular problems; secondly to examine in more detail the ways in which the legal system has responded to those problems; finally to consider whether that response is satisfactory.

What features of MMCs give rise to particular problems?

MMCs give rise to a number of problems for the legal system. Before identifying those features of MMCs that are responsible for those problems, we should be clear about whose concerns we should aim to address. Most obvious are the concerns of the courts in the efficient administration of justice. These are of paramount importance, and should certain factors present in MMCs impede the pursuit of that objective that would be a significant matter. Yet no less important are the concerns of those who allege they have been injured by a medical product. If victims of mass medical torts are denied access to justice that would tend to frustrate the pursuit of the central objectives of tort law: compensation and deterrence. On one side of the coin we find that many who suffer serious injury have to fall back on the bare minimum support provided by the social security system. On the other side we find that the wrongdoing of mass tortfeasors goes unchecked. To the extent that tort law is justified by reference to the incentives it gives people to take care not to harm others, that "deterrence" objective is undermined if those others are unable to enforce their right to tort damages. Furthermore, looking beyond the particular concerns of tort law, it may be that the lack of effective access to remedies may result in a general alienation on the part of the population at large from the courts and other institutions of government.[13] These considerations suggest that any analysis of the problems presented by MMCs should look at the problems facing plaintiffs in such cases as well as those facing the courts.

Having defined our terms of reference in such a way, we can now seek to identify and examine those features of MMCs that are the source of the problems encountered by courts and plaintiffs.

The problem of numbers

Medical products manufactured with a defect in their design may well inflict injuries on vast numbers of people. The Dalkon shield, an intra-uterine contraceptive device, is alleged to have injured over 200 000 women worldwide, some 3000–4000 of them in Britain.[14] Cases of this sort raise concerns of judicial economy: "Trying 1500 cases together is much cheaper than trying 1500 cases separately." Sir John Donaldson's words, uttered in the course of the Opren litigation,[15] point to a simple truth: where related cases raise common issues, it is a waste of time and money to try these issues again and again in separate trials. Indeed, one judge has been moved to describe the needless re-examination of common questions as "a scandal to the administration of justice".[16] Looking across the Atlantic, it was the same concern that prompted Judge Spencer Williams (a Californian judge writing extra-judicially) to pose the following rhetorical question:

> "Is it effective or efficient use of juridical resources to subject a judge to the tedious and frustrating task of presiding over identical lawsuits, or even to distribute these cases throughout the court system to occupy calendars in many courts?"[17]

In addition to financial considerations, the prospect of inconsistent verdicts and concomitant uncertainty in the law arising from the separate trial of identical issues give the legal system cause to look for some sort of special procedure to deal with the problem of numbers. Treating like cases alike is a prerequisite for a just system of law. This was recognised by the Australian Law Reform

Commission in its call for the introduction of a grouped representative procedure (a class action in all but name) in the federal courts in Australia. Commenting on the fact that Victorian and West Australian courts had reached different conclusions as to liability in the asbestos litigation, the commission pointed out how the decisions tended to undermine public confidence in the legal system: "Such inconsistencies can result in courts being seen as inefficient and unfair."[18]

The problem of cost

We have already noted how court resources might be drained purely and simply on account of the fact that medical products often harm large numbers of people. The problem of cost, however, also rears its head quite independently of the problem of numbers. This is because MMCs typically raise issues that make litigation exceedingly costly. This expense can be attributed to two hurdles that stand between the plaintiff and success. In the first place, the plaintiff must establish that the medical product was the cause of her injury.[19] Where that injury is typically associated with a particular medical product, the causation hurdle is readily surmounted. An example of this is the rare vaginal cancer found in the offspring of women who had taken the drug diethylstilboestrol (DES) during pregnancy.[20] By contrast, where the individual plaintiff's condition is one that might have been produced by any one of a number of factors, she will have to rule out each of those other alternative causes. Often the causal processes in question are obscure and can only be illuminated, if at all, with the aid of detailed clinical and epidemiological evidence. It was this hurdle that was the downfall of the plaintiff in *Loveday* v. *Renton*,[21] the test case brought in relation to the use of the pertussis (whooping cough) vaccine in which it was held that there was insufficient evidence that the vaccine could cause brain damage.

In the second place, the plaintiff must prove either that the product was negligently manufactured or supplied (for a claim in the tort of negligence)[22] or alternatively that the product was defective (for a claim under the Consumer Protection Act 1987).[23] This is a particularly difficult task in the typical MMC. In such a case, it is rare for the plaintiff to be able to point to a simple malfunction in the manufacturing process of the nature of the decomposed snail that is left in the bottle of ginger beer. This is commonly termed a "manufacturing defect" and raises in itself a very strong presumption both that the manufacturer was negligent and that the product was defective. In an MMC, however, the plaintiff will generally have to establish that the design of the product was defective (in a claim in negligence as well as a claim under the Consumer Protection Act) as it is the fact that all the products were defective that explains why so many people were injured. This calls for a complex cost–benefit analysis. The questions raised in such cases – what was the risk of harmful side-effects resulting from use of the product? was running that risk acceptable in view of the benefits that product might bring? – go far beyond everyday experience and call for the evidence of experts who must sift through pile upon pile of documentation to find out who did what, when, and with what knowledge.

All in all, gathering and making sense of evidence relating to causation, negligence and defectiveness is a hugely costly exercise – one that is beyond the means of most individual litigants. Confirmation of this view, and an indication of the scale of the task facing victims of mass medical torts, was given by Hirst J in his review of the Opren litigation:

> "I wish to stress certain special features of this unique case. It has involved the discovery and inspection of millions of documents, together with a huge effort of assessment and scrutiny by several categories of scientific, medical, pharmaceutical and legal experts. No single plaintiff could conceivably have mounted such a colossal enterprise on his or her own."[24]

The problem of ignorance

Ignorance, like cost, can represent a substantial barrier in the way of those worthy of compensation for injuries arising out of the use of medical products. Victims may be ignorant of their rights in particular circumstances or of how to enforce them. In some cases, they may even be ignorant of the fact that they have been injured at all or may fail to link their condition to the use of a particular medical product. This may well be so, for instance, where the injury in question takes the form of delayed side-effects from dangerous pharmaceutical products that cannot be traced to particular medication without expert assistance.[25] In such cases, the victim may attribute her condition to natural causes rather than link it with use of the dangerous product. Over and above this "access to justice" concern is the fear that potential claimants, unaware of the progress of other related actions, might unnecessarily relitigate the same issues. This would conflict with the goal of efficiency in the administration of justice and import uncertainty and possibly inconsistency into the law.

Judicial responses to the problems raised by MMCs

To the present day, courts facing mass medical cases have had to muddle by within the constraints of existing procedures provided by the Rules of the Supreme Court (set out in the "White Book"). In so doing, they have declared an intention to be "as flexible and adaptable as possible in the application of existing procedures with a view to reaching decisions quickly and economically".[26] A commitment to the *ad hoc* resolution of procedural problems is not, however, a sound basis for multi-party litigation. As Steyn J pointed out in the course of litigation concerning the medical product Myodil, "Our system of civil justice ought, for the benefits of parties involved in group litigation, to prescribe at least in outline the procedures to be adopted."[27] He suggested that the best way forward might be by a "gradualistic approach": rather than opt for wholesale legislative reform, a guide could be published so as "not ... to produce a procedural straitjacket but to set out in outline the alternative procedures which are available, and the range of the court's powers".[28] The Supreme Court Procedure Committee has now published such a guide, produced by a working party consisting of Judge Bowsher QC, Andrew Smith QC and Rodger Pannone. The guide lent its seal of approval to the various ways in which existing procedures have been shaped to meet the demands of MMCs and it is to these procedures that we now turn.

Organising the plaintiffs

Before claimants in a multi-party case can reap the benefits of the special procedures outlined below, they must organise themselves into a group. The first difficulty they will face in doing so is to identify all those in a similar position to themselves who might want to join, and spread the costs of the group. The other claimants may be located across the country: some will already have started legal action, others will not. To help plaintiffs get in contact with other interested parties, the Law Society set up in the aftermath of the Zeebrugge Ferry disaster a disaster coordination service after particular encouragement from the Consumers Association.[29] The service is currently dealing with the benzodiazepine tranquilliser addiction, myodoxil X-ray dye and steroids actions. Its method of operation is immediately following a disaster to issue a press release to the national press and media and to advertise a "hot-line" telephone number. Members of the public who contact the service are directed to a suitable solicitor. Solicitors who use the hot-line are given details of other firms dealing with similar cases. The *Guide for Use in Group Actions* suggests that solicitors concerned then form themselves into a solicitors' group and within a few weeks appoint a coordinating or steering committee comprising usually five or six firms of solicitors. This committee is entrusted with the task of supervising the litigation and of supplying other members of the solicitors' group with information and guidance about the progress of the case.

Choosing a form of procedure

English law, unlike that of the United States, knows no so-called "class action".[30] At first glance, the representative action under Order 15 rule 12 of the Rules of the Supreme Court is somewhat similar. In cases where "numerous persons have the same interest in any proceedings", the rules allow one of them to conduct the proceedings as the representative of the others. However, the representative action differs from the paradigmatic class action in that the result of a representative action binds all members of the represented group whether they like it or not. In a class action, claimants are generally allowed to exercise their choice to prosecute their cases independently by opting out of, or declining to opt in to, the action.

In England, the representative action has, as yet, played no role in mass medical cases. This is primarily because of doubts as to whether plaintiffs claiming damages on their own behalf can be said to have the requisite "same interest" in the proceedings. Successive editions of the "White Book" have cited the leading case of *Markt & Co. Ltd* v. *Knight Steamship Co. Ltd*[31] as authority for the proposition that, in the words of Fletcher Moulton LJ, "no representative action can lie where the sole relief sought is damages, because they have to be proved separately in the case of each plaintiff ... ".[32] In fact, only Fletcher Moulton LJ of the majority of the Court of Appeal based his decision on this ground.[33] In a more recent case, *Prudential Assurance Co. Ltd* v. *Newman Industries Ltd*,[34] Vinelott J showed a willingness to take a wider view of the availability of the representative action. He held that it was possible to use the Order 15 rule 12 procedure to enable shareholders in a company to obtain a declaration that they, and the other shareholders (not themselves parties to the action), were entitled to damages from the directors of the company in relation to an alleged conspiracy by the directors. This use of the Order 15, rule 12, procedure has been regarded as creating a declaratory class action. It would seem possible to apply the same approach to MMCs. In the first instance, one of the victims might seek a declaration that the product in question was defective and that the defect was capable of producing injuries of the type actually sustained. Subsequently, the other victims could go to court separately to prove that their injuries were in fact caused by the defect and to establish the extent of their individual loss. Alternatively, the parties might agree on a compensation scheme under which the appropriate payment for each individual would be determined out of court. Be this as it may, the possibility of a declaratory class action (falling short of the payment of damages) has not been pursued in MMCs in England.

Instead, the English approach to MMCs is centred upon the test case. The standard procedure involves two stages. At the first, all the cases are brought together before the same judge; at the second stage, certain of the cases are selected to go forward as lead actions while the other actions are stayed pending the outcome of those actions. In relation to the first stage, it is the usual practice to bring all the cases together by informal means rather than by relying on the rules relating to the procedures of joinder or consolidation. Joinder is the process of starting one action under the same writ in the name of all plaintiffs and is dealt with under Rules of the Supreme Court Order 15, rule 4. This may be more convenient and less costly than having each plaintiff start an action separately. As the *Guide for Use in Group Actions* points out, "To issue one writ on behalf of 1001 plaintiffs instead of one writ on behalf of each of those plaintiffs produces a saving of £70 000 in court fees for the writ alone and a further saving of at least £10 000 for each interlocutory summons later issued."[35] In multi-incident cases, however, a multiplicity of writs will be almost inevitable: individual plaintiffs will invariably be ignorant of others in the same position, or may be reluctant to switch from their own solicitor to the firm handling the joint litigation, while their solicitors may have advised them to issue a writ as soon as possible so as to avoid problems with limitation of actions. The formal legal procedure to group together a large number of actions that have already been started is known as consolidation. Where there is a multiplicity of actions, the courts have a wide discretion to "consolidate" those actions wherever it considers it desirable to deal with them together.[36] However, it is more usual for the Lord Chief Justice to proceed informally by nominating one judge to take over the whole of the conduct of a group of actions.

Generally, the judge will be a High Court judge based in London and, as claimants in the group will invariably have issued writs in district registries around the country, it will be necessary for them to apply to have their cases transferred to the Central Office of the High Court in London. To alert the claimants to this, the Lord Chief Justice may issue a Practice Note advising the parties of the need to do so in order to facilitate the handling of the litigation.[37] Once proceedings are placed under the supervision of a single judge who is well acquainted with the case, a number of opportunities for reducing expense open up. A good example of the steps that might be taken is to be found in "the Opren scheme", devised by Hirst J and the parties appearing before him in the Opren litigation:

> "Great efforts are being made at the suggestion of the Court, and with the willing co-operation of all parties, to minimise expense, for example by making use of short two-page specimen pleadings or schedules, cross-referenced to the very long and complicated Master Statement of Claim and the two Master Defences of the respective group of defendants; and by organising one single discovery process to cover as many actions as possible."[38]

The second stage of the usual English procedure is to select a number of the claims to go forward as test cases or lead actions while proceedings in the others are stayed by an order of the court.[39] The selection will be designed to make sure that all generic issues are the subject of judicial decision for the benefit of the other claimants. For these purposes, the term "generic issues" covers not only those issues that affect all plaintiffs in the group but also those issues that affect a reasonably sizeable class of plaintiffs. The test case procedure has advantages for all concerned, as is borne out by the fact that "over several years past, employers and trade unions have co-operated in selecting plaintiffs in trades union financed litigation concerning industrial injuries to obtain judicial decisions on the appropriate damages over a range of cases to help legal advisers on both sides reach settlements of other cases".[40] In the consolidated Opren litigation, the plan was to take certain lead cases to trial on the large number of issues on liability that were common to all the individual actions, in particular those relating to the development of the drug, its testing, and the evaluation of the possible side-effects. Hirst J explained that the lead plaintiffs would have to be "suitably representative of the various categories into which Opren plaintiffs can conveniently be divided, having regard in particular to the plaintiffs' medical history, to represent the various different aspects relevant to the issues of liability".[41] In the event, the actions were settled before they came to trial.

Test cases do not in strict law bind the other plaintiffs in the test case scheme on questions of fact. This is potentially a major drawback of the test case procedure, as it seems to allow common questions addressed in the test cases to be relitigated by those (be they plaintiff or defendant) whose actions have been stayed and who are not satisfied by the outcome of the test case.[42] This multiplicity of actions would be an unnecessary burden on the courts, risk inconsistency and place additional barriers in the way of the tort victim seeking compensation. However, it is possible for those involved in the litigation to give an undertaking to be bound by the result of the test cases. Even in the absence of such an undertaking, it may be that the court will use its jurisdiction to strike out claims or defences as an abuse of process in order to prevent relitigation of points determined in a test case. Although the courts are not prepared fully to define the circumstances in which relitigation might be regarded as an abuse of process, one such circumstance might be where the plaintiff has joined a test case scheme and, having had an opportunity to be heard on the selection of test plaintiffs, has not objected to the selection made.[43] An example of this is *Godfrey* v. *Department of Health and Social Security*, an unreported decision of Stuart-Smith J in chambers.[44] The case was part of the litigation arising out of the use of the pertussis (whooping cough) vaccine in which it was alleged that various doctors, nurses and health authorities had been negligent in giving injections to young children with the result that they had suffered serious brain damage. Stuart-Smith J was given the task of overseeing the many cases in which proceedings had been started. He decided to adopt a test case strategy in order to resolve the question of whether the vaccine was capable of causing brain damage (the issue of "generic causation") and accordingly stayed all the actions but for one, *Loveday* v. *Renton*,[45] in which he directed that there should be trial of the issue of causation as a preliminary issue. After a lengthy trial, in the course of which no expense was spared on behalf of the legally aided plaintiff, the judge reached the conclusion that the case on causation was not proven. Subsequently, the plaintiff Godfrey sought to bring a similar action, albeit against a different defendant. On the defendant's application, Stuart-Smith J struck out the action under Rules of the Supreme Court Order 18, rule 9, as an abuse of the process of the court, the action being an attempt to relitigate the same issue in the absence of fresh evidence that bore materially on the issue of causation. Despite this decision, the precise scope of the court's power to strike out actions for abuse of process in this sphere remains uncertain. This may well provoke disputes which the *Guide for Use in Group Actions* suggests might be avoided if the judge were to make an express order in advance of the trial of the test actions that parties to all other actions in the scheme should be bound by the findings of fact in those actions.[46]

Financing the action[47]

Current judicial practice is to order that the costs of pursuing a multi-party medical action be shared equally between all the members of the plaintiff group, whether or not the particular member's case is selected to go forward as a lead action. A costs order of this sort was made by Hirst J in the course of the Opren litigation and approved by the Court of Appeal.[48] Previously, for instance in the Thalidomide and Primodos litigation, the plaintiffs pursuing the lead actions had borne all the costs of the litigation without contribution from those not party to the actions.[49] As the test case plaintiffs were invariably funded by legal aid, this meant that absent members of the plaintiff group got a "free ride" at the expense of the Legal Aid Fund, irrespective of whether they themselves were entitled to legal aid. The Opren decision finally put paid to this practice.

The Court of Appeal pointed out that this change of approach was required by concerns of fairness, not only to the defendant who will rarely be able to recover costs from the Legal Aid Fund,[50] but also to the plaintiffs.[51] In the case of the latter, there was a risk of injustice stemming from the fact that the Legal Aid Fund might be required to "claw back" some of the costs incurred in the lead actions from the damages awarded to the test plaintiffs. This claw-back provision, termed the "statutory charge", comes into operation whenever the costs incurred by the Fund exceed those recovered from the defendant. This may be the case if the defendant has no money or the Fund has to incur further expense in making the defendant pay. Even if this is not so, the court will only require the defendant to pay those costs that it has assessed as reasonable: these "taxed" costs are almost always less than the costs which have been incurred by the plaintiffs in prosecuting their cases to a successful conclusion. Furthermore, a number of interlocutory hearings might have been necessary as the test cases were brought to full trial and, if the plaintiffs were unsuccessful in these, they might be ordered to pay the defendant's costs in them. These considerations led Sir John Donaldson MR in the Opren case to emphasise that the claw-back provisions would inevitably be called into operation: "there will always be a shortfall, which may be very large".[52] In his view, there was a very real danger that the damages awarded to the plaintiffs in the lead action would be swallowed up by the Legal Aid Fund:

> "None of them would ever get a penny piece by way of compensation. Anything which the defendants were ordered to pay in respect of damages, costs and interest would be totally absorbed in paying their own costs. This would be a grossly unfair situation . . ."[53]

Even now that it is clear that the courts will not allow any one plaintiff to bear a liability to more than a proportionate share of the total costs, the costs factor remains a significant deterrent. In the Opren litigation, the costs would have been shared between some 1500 plaintiffs, each of whom would pay only 66p per £1000 of costs incurred. Yet when the court ruled that the absent group members could not get a free ride on the backs of the legally aided test plaintiffs, the 500 or so of them who were not entitled to legal aid announced their intention to discontinue their actions. It was only the generosity of a millionaire, Mr Godfrey Bradman, in offering to underwrite the costs of their claim that persuaded them not to do so.[54]

The fear that tort victims might be deterred from seeking compensation has prompted law review bodies in other jurisdictions to advocate reform of cost rules in cases of this sort. They suggest the replacement of the current "two-way"costs rule (under which the losing side must generally reimburse the winner for its costs) with a "no-way"[55] or, more radically, a "one-way"[56] costs regime. A "no-way" costs rule – standard in the United States – effectively entails the abolition of awards of costs *inter partes*: each side pays its own costs no matter who wins. A "one-way" rule as to costs would allow the plaintiffs, if successful, to recover their costs from the defendant but would shield them from any liability for costs if they lost. A reform of this "heads I win, tails you lose" nature seems unjustly to discriminate against defendants. However, its proponents argue that this is a price worth paying to avoid the greater injustice now done to large numbers of people who suffer loss and who, due to economic barriers, have no effective remedy. They argue further that the potential for injustice is palliated by the fact that defendants are likely to be large corporations or public bodies.[57] In fact, just such a costs regime already operates on a limited scale in Britain where a non-legally aided defendant generally has no claim against the Legal Aid Fund in respect of its costs incurred in warding off a claim by an assisted plaintiff.[58] Both a "one-way" and a "no-way" costs regime would improve the position of tort plaintiffs by taking away the fear that they might be held liable for the defendant's costs. However, reform along these lines would leave them liable for a share of the costs incurred by their own team of lawyers in litigating the action.

To reduce the costs barrier further, many argue that reform of solicitor and client costs should accompany reform of costs between the parties. This has resulted in pressure to accept, at least in the context of multi-party actions, the legality of "contingency fees", so named as they are paid only if the outcome of the case is successful.[59] At present, solicitors in England are not entitled to take on cases on this basis. Although no longer criminal as maintenance or champerty,[60] such agreements are unenforceable[61] and unethical.[62] However, under the Courts and Legal Services Act 1990, the Lord Chancellor is given the power to make orders allowing use of "conditional fee arrangements" in appropriate circumstances.[63] He has yet to make use of this power, though the *Guide for Use in Group Actions* suggests that, when brought into effect, the provision is likely to be relevant to group actions.[64]

Although existing costs rules may be tailored to reduce the potential costs exposure of victims of mass torts, increased public funding may prove ultimately to be the only way of ensuring that multi-party actions furnish these victims with an effective remedy. This view is attracting growing support in Britain. In 1988, during the debates in the House of Lords on the Legal Aid Bill, the Law Society suggested (unsuccessfully) an amendment designed to alleviate some of the funding problems revealed by the Opren litigation.[65] By the terms of this amendment, where there was judicial certification of a group action, the Legal Aid Board would grant free representation to all those within the group.

The arguments for public funding of multi-party actions have now been examined by the Legal Aid Board itself in the course of its efforts to develop special arrangements for the handling of such actions.[66] These special arrangements will be implemented by making use of the power, granted to the Legal Aid Board by section 4 of the Legal Aid Act 1988, to make contracts with a firm of solicitors to provide legal aid representation in civil matters.[67] The idea is that in multi-party cases involving personal injury the Board may enter into such contracts with a lead firm of solicitors who will undertake the generic work on behalf of all claimants; the role of other solicitors will be limited to liaising directly with their clients and dealing with the special issues raised only by their individual cases. Once these arrangements are in place, it is proposed that legal aid will only be available to claimants within the arrangements. In its report to the Lord Chancellor of September 1991, the Legal Aid Board expressed no concluded view on the question of whether all those involved in the multi-party litigation should be eligible to take advantage of the special arrangements, irrespective of whether they passed the means test that generally governs the availability of legal aid. The Board left consideration of this matter to the Lord Chancellor's Department, which is currently midway through a major review of eligibility.[68] However, in an earlier consultation paper, the Board had expressed its initial view that legal aid should be extended to all, regardless of income but subject to the payment of a contribution in appropriate cases. In taking this view, the Board was influenced by the fact that the costs of pursuing an action of this kind might make it impracticable for all but the wealthiest non-assisted claimants to litigate and the likelihood that the marginal costs of pursuing most of the additional cases would be small.[69] The consultation paper gives no details of how the contribution provisions would operate and there remains the risk that mass tort victims might be deterred from litigating their claims even by a liability to a proportionate share of the costs. A reasonable compromise solution, favoured by the National Consumer Council,[70] would be to limit the amount of the contribution to an arbitrary figure of, say, £1000.

Conclusion

Courts and lawyers have shown great ingenuity in adapting existing legal procedures for use in MMCs. Without such ingenuity, the procedures might have buckled under the extraordinary pressures put on them. The result has been a considerable saving of cost for both the courts and the parties. Yet, the adoption of a series of *ad hoc* solutions is not a wholly satisfactory manner of dealing with the modern phenomenon of the MMC. As was pointed out above, lawyers can only be expected to handle these cases effectively if given a procedural framework within which to work.[71] The provision of a guide to group litigation is only a partial answer to this problem, for the extent of the court's jurisdiction outside the formalities of the "White Book" remains in doubt and the risk of a successful challenge to the procedure adopted might be an effective weapon in the hands of a corporate defendant in the out-of-court settlement process.[72]

More fundamentally, we must question whether existing legal procedures satisfactorily address the special problems presented by mass torts. We have seen that the development of the test case procedure has enabled the courts to deal with a large number of claims without unnecessary relitigation of common questions. This keeps costs to a minimum for both courts and plaintiffs and seeks to ensure that like cases are treated alike. The problem of numbers, therefore, has been addressed with some degree of success. When it comes to the problem of cost, however, the picture is less satisfactory. As the Opren litigation reveals, non-legally aided victims of medical products may be deterred from pursuing their legal remedies by the fear of costs. One can only hope that the Legal Aid Board's special procedure for multi-party actions, implemented recently, is made available to all, regardless of means, though subject to payment of a contribution in appropriate cases.

This leaves the problem of ignorance. Of all the problems raised by MMCs, this has received the least attention. Yet it is far from insignificant. Ignorance of group proceedings might cause the victims concerned to miss the deadline date for joining the group. Where this occurs, they might be precluded from suing independently, either as a matter of law (e.g. because they fall outside the limitation periods) or because they cannot bear the costs of the action on their own. Even if they do proceed with their own actions, this only results in undesirable and avoidable relitigation. The chief reason why the problem of ignorance has yet to be resolved is that the current MMC procedure requires those seeking compensation to take affirmative action to "opt in" to the group action. Unless victims of mass medical torts have knowledge of their right to opt in, that right is worth nothing to lia[73] and Ontario[74] to advocate special new procedures for multi-party actions in which all potential plaintiffs are bound by the result of an action brought on their behalf unless they exercise their right to "opt out". As a corollary to this, they also advocated that procedures be adopted for the purpose of giving "notice" (for instance by press advertisement or television broadcast) of the litigation to those that might fall within the plaintiff class.[75]

A more extreme approach is suggested by the representative procedure under Rules of the Supreme Court Order 15, rule 12. Uniquely amongst existing English procedures, there is no need for members of the represented class to opt in to the action. However, there is no opportunity to opt out of a representative action either: all class members are bound whether they like it or not. In other words, membership of the represented class is mandatory. This may be regarded as going too far in response to the problems of mass torts and as requiring too great a sacrifice of the individual's right to control the course of her own litigation. Those that can afford to do so should be free to opt out of the group litigation and to bring their own action. Of course, many will be precluded from doing so by financial constraints. However, in such cases, the *de facto* limitation of their right to conduct their own litigation should be counterbalanced by the provision of procedural safeguards adequate to protect their interests. Wherever members of the plaintiff class are absent from the trial of common questions, there is always the danger that the representative plaintiff might conduct the litigation and the settlement process in order to advance her own interest at the expense of the represented plaintiffs. In spite of this, the procedure under Rules of the Supreme Court Order 15 rule 12 gives represented plaintiffs no right to give voice to concerns about the conduct of the case, nor does it require that any settlement be submitted for judicial approval. Such concerns seem to have been in the forefront of Fletcher Moulton LJ's mind as he sought to limit the scope of the representative action in the *Markt* case: "I can conceive of no excuse for allowing any one shipper to conduct litigation on behalf of another without his leave, and yet so as to bind him."[76] In sum, the mandatory nature of the representative action and the lack of any framework for safeguarding the interests of group members make it an unsuitable procedure for dealing with MMCs.

In view of the deficiencies of existing procedures, the time has now come to introduce a class action procedure for use in MMCs. The new procedure would be able to confront head-on the problems posed by such cases. In particular, it would contain provision for public funding through the Legal Aid Fund, which would benefit all plaintiffs whether or not they were entitled to legal aid (though perhaps eligibility would depend on payment of a contribution in appropriate cases). To deal with the problem of ignorance, the procedure would treat all potential claimants as bound by the result of the group proceedings, unless they chose to opt out of those proceedings, and would authorise judges to require the parties to publicise the proceedings, for example by taking out advertisements in the press or on television. In this way, the procedure would give individual claimants the knowledge necessary to enforce their rights through the group action and prevent unnecessary relitigation.

Notes and references

1. The account that follows draws heavily upon the judgment of Hidden J in *Nash* v. *Eli Lilly & Co.* [1991] 2 Med LR 169; see also Mildred and Pannone, "Class actions" in M. Powers and N. Harris (eds.), *Medical Negligence* (1990) at 12.75–12.87.
2. See generally J.G. Fleming, *The American Tort Process* (1988,

Oxford University Press), ch. 4: "the civil jury in tort litigation has become the darling of plaintiffs and the scourge of defendants" (at 103).

3. See generally C. Munro and H. Teff, *Thalidomide: The Legal Aftermath* (1976).
4. *Davies* v. *Eli Lilly & Co.* (1987) 137 NLJ 1183.
5. *Davies* v. *Eli Lilly & Co.* (unreported, Queen's Bench Division, 14 January 1988).
6. *R* v. *Legal Aid Area no. 8 (Northern) Appeal Committee, Ex parte Angell* (1990) *The Times* 13 March.
7. *Beal* v. *Eli Lilly & Co.* (unreported, Queen's Bench Division, 30 March 1988).
8. *Davies* v. *Eli Lilly & Co.* (unreported, Queen's Bench Division, 22 July 1987).
9. *Davies* v. *Eli Lilly & Co.* [1987] 1 WLR 428.
10. *Nash* v. *Eli Lilly & Co.* [1991] 2 Med LR 169.
11. Ibid at 174.
12. See generally JG Fleming, op cit supra note 2, ch. 7.
13. Ontario Law Reform Commission, *Report on Class Actions* (1982), p. 125 (hereafter "Ontario Report").
14. See R.M. Dias and B.S. Markesinis, *Tort Law* (2nd edn. 1989) p. 3.
15. *Davies* v. *Eli Lilly & Co. Ltd* [1987] 3 All ER 94 at 100.
16. *Amos* v. *Chadwick* (1978) 9 Ch D 459 at 462 per Jessel MR.
17. S. Williams, "Mass tort class actions: going, going, gone" (1983) 98 FRD 323 at 325.
18. Report of the Law Reform Commission (Cth) [Australia], *Grouped Proceedings in the Federal Court* (ALRC 46; 1988), para. 66 (hereafter "Australian Report").
19. See generally J. Stapleton, *Disease and the Compensation Debate* (1986), ch. 3; Newdick, "Strict liability for defective drugs in the pharmaceutical industry" (1985) 101 LQR 405 at 420–30.
20. J. Stapleton, op cit at 34–5.
21. [1990] 1 Med. LR 117; for an example of these issues arising outside the context of the MMC, see *Hotson* v. *East Berkshire Area Health Authority* [1987] AC 750.
22. See generally J. Stapleton, op cit ch. 4.
23. See generally Newdick, op cit at 409–20.
24. *Davies* v. *Eli Lilly & Co.* (1987) 137 NLJ 1183 at 1184 per Hirst J.
25. Ontario Report, supra note 13 at 127–8; see further *Nash* v. *Eli Lilly & Co.* [1991] 2 Med LR 169 (dealing with limitation problems in such cases).
26. *Davies* v. *Eli Lilly & Co.* [1987] 3 All ER 94 at 96 per Sir John Donaldson MR.
27. *Chrzanowska* v. *Glaxo Laboratories Ltd* [1990] 1 Med LR 385 at 386.

28. Ibid.
29. See *Guide for Use in Group Actions*, Appendix 1; also "In the news" (1992) 142 NLJ 114.
30. Even in the United States, courts have been reluctant to apply the class action procedure contained in the Federal Rules of Civil Procedure (Rule 23) to MMCs: see, for example, *In re Northern District of California "Dalkon Shield" IUD Product Liability Litigation* (1981) 526 F Supp 887, (1982) 693 F 2d 847. See generally J. G. Fleming, op cit, supra note 2 at 237–51.
31. [1910] 2 QB 1021.
32. Ibid at 1040; see also *Chrzanowska* v. *Glaxo Laboratories Ltd* [1990] 1 Med LR 385 at 386.
33. The other judge in the majority, Vaughan Williams LJ, based his decision on the somewhat narrower ground that the claims lacked a "common purpose".
34. [1979] 3 All ER 507; see also *The Irish Rowan* [1989] 3 All ER 853 at 864, 868 and 876.
35. p. 18.
36. RSC Order 4, rule 9.
37. See the Practice Note given by the Lord Chief Justice on 6 December 1990 recording the nomination of Ian Kennedy J to monitor the progress of the benzodiazepine litigation (reprinted in Appendix 2 of the *Guide For Use in Group Actions*).
38. *Davies* v. *Eli Lilly & Co.* (Queen's Bench Division, 23 July 1986).
39. Again under RSC order 4, rule 9.
40. *Guide for Use in Group Actions* at 21; see, for example, *Thompson* v. *Smith Shiprepairers Ltd* [1984] 2 WLR 522.
41. *Davies* v. *Eli Lilly & Co.* (Queen's Bench Division, 23 July 1986).
42. Australian Report, op cit, paras 54–6; Ontario Report, op cit, at 87–8.
43. *Ashmore* v. *British Coal Corp.* [1990] 2 All ER 981 at 987–8.
44. Queen's Bench Division, 25 July 1988, unreported.
45. [1990] 1 Med LR 117.
46. p. 21.
47. See generally J.G. Fleming, op cit, supra note 2, ch. 6.
48. *Davies* v. *Eli Lilly & Co.* [1987] 3 All ER 94.
49. See Mildred and Pannone, op cit, supra note 1 at 12.78.
50. Legal Aid Act 1988, s. 18 limits the recovery of costs from the Fund by an unassisted party to cases in which that party "will suffer severe financial hardship" unless payment is made.
51. *Davies* v. *Eli Lilly & Co.* [1987] 3 All ER 94 at 100.
52. Ibid at 98.
53. Ibid at 98.
54. National Consumer Council, *Group Actions: Learning from Opren* (1988) at 29–30.
55. Ontario Report supra, note 13 at 706.

56. Thirty-Sixth Report of the Law Reform Committee of South Australia Relating to Class Actions (1977) at 8.
57. Ibid.
58. Legal Aid Act 1988, s. 18; the contribution of an unsuccessful assisted plaintiff to the costs of the defendant is limited to such sum as is reasonable having regard to all the circumstances: s. 17. See also note 49 supra.
59. Australian Report, supra note 18 at 293; Ontario Report, supra note 13 at 713–16.
60. Criminal Law Act 1967, ss. 13 and 14.
61. Solicitors Act 1974, s. 59(2)(b).
62. See *Wallersteiner* v. *Moir (No. 2)* [1975] QB 373.
63. Section 58; for a discussion see Swanson, "The importance of conditional fee agreements (1991) 11 OJLS 193.
64. At 28.
65. See National Consumer Council, *Group Actions: Learning from Opren* at 30.
66. Legal Aid Board, *Report on Proposals to the Lord Chancellor Relating to the Legal Aid Aspects of Multi-party Actions* (1991).
67. See Civil Legal Aid (General Amendment) Regulations 1992 SI 1992 No 590.
68. Ibid at 31.
69. Legal Aid Board, *Consultation Paper on Multi-party Actions* (1990) para. 24.
70. *Group Actions: Learning from Opren* at 35–6; see also Mildred and Pannone, supra note 1, paras 12.95–12.100.
71. Supra at text accompanying note 49.
72. See Mildred and Pannone, supra note 1, para. 12.77. The inequality of bargaining power between the protagonists in this process is well-documented: see especially H. Genn, *Hard Bargaining* (1987).
73. Supra note 18 at 118–22.
74. Supra note 13 at 484–85.
75. Supra note 18 at 182 and note 13 at 516.
76. [1910] 2 QB 1021 at 1040.

The medical and legal response to post-traumatic stress disorder*

Michael Napier

In 1987 Rodger Pannone described the differences between the so-called "creeping disaster" (for example drug cases such as Opren or the benzodiazepines) and the "instant disaster" (e.g. transport accidents).[1] This chapter almost exclusively relates to instant disasters.

Six possible definitions of a disaster are:

1. *Shorter Oxford Dictionary*: "Anything ruinous or distressing that befalls; a sudden or great misfortune or mishap; a calamity."
2. *Chambers 20th Century Dictionary*: "A sudden and great misfortune."
3. *Longmans English Dictionary*: "A sudden or great misfortune, especially a sudden calamity bringing great damage, loss or estruction."
4. *The Cranfield Disaster Preparedness Centre*: "Any situation

* Editor's note: Mr Napier's chapter was presented as a Lent Lecture at King's College on 4 March 1991 and at a meeting of the Medico-Legal Society on 14 February 1991. The text of the latter was published in (1991) 59 *Medico-Legal Journal* 157 and is reproduced here with permission.

Choices and Decisions in Health Care. Edited by A. Grubb.

resulting from natural or man made catastrophe demanding total integration of the rescue, emergency services and life support systems available to those responsible for the affected areas together with the communication and transportation resources required to support relief operations."

5. "A situation arising with or without warning, causing or threatening death, injury or serious disruption to normal life, for numbers of people in excess of those which can be dealt with by the public and Social Services operating under normal conditions and requiring the special mobilisation and organisation of those services."
6. "Any incident where there is one more casualty than the emergency service can cope with."

The sixth definition has the benefit of simplicity. It talks of "casualty", and it is the casualty to people that we are talking about.

In a disaster there is frequently a special type of casualty that may be described as "non-physical injury". The courts used to call it "nervous shock", a term which has now been disapproved and replaced by "psychiatric injury", or sometimes "psychiatric illness or damage".[2] These are "umbrella" terms embracing a family of psychiatric illnesses, of which the now well-known condition of post-traumatic stress disorder (PTSD) is but one. Five years ago, PTSD was unknown to lawyers in the UK and it was understood, as far as I am aware, only by a few psychiatrists and psychologists. Today it is a term which is widely and quite loosely used to mean shock sustained in any accident and particularly in a disaster. Just as journalists enthusiastically talk about "class actions" (which is a concept unknown to English law, but they always talk about it after a disaster),* they now talk about PTSD as part of their regular vocabulary. UK lawyers now look for PTSD as a matter of course when assessing their clients' compensation in a whole variety of accident situations, not necessarily confined to disasters. Today there are even several private clinics springing up specialising in the counselling and treatment of PTSD and there are calls for similar facilities to be provided more widely by the National Health Service.

So how was it that PTSD came to be recognised? It was initially

---

* Editor's note: see the chapter by Ken Oliphant in this volume.

described in the United States following research on Vietnam war veterans. The American Psychiatric Association, in its 1980 edition of the *Diagnostic and Statistical Manual of Mental Disorders* (known as DSM III R), listed the features of PTSD (see Appendix 1) and the diagnostic criteria, (see Appendix 2).

Similar descriptions to those found in DSM III R now appear in the *International Classification of Diseases* (known as ICD), published by the World Health Organization.

Professor John Gunn who, with some of his colleagues at the Institute of Psychiatry, has given valuable help in assessing and reporting on victims of disasters, believes that DSM III R is more frequently referred to than ICD9, so it is quite legitimate for psychiatrists preparing medico-legal reports to rely on the DSM III R criteria. Professor Gunn also regards the recognition of PTSD in recent years as a good illustration of the way in which diagnostic categories in medicine emerge and crystallise.

The medical literature supporting the gradual recognition of PTSD begins as far back as 1917, with a paper by Mott in the *British Medical Journal* entitled "Mental hygiene and shell shock during and after the war".[3] The military emphasis reappears in 1943, with a paper by Symons, also in the *British Medical Journal*,[4] under the title "The human response to flying stress", and in 1949 a paper by Swank in the *Journal of Nervous and Mental Diseases* describing combat exhaustion.[5]

There were more papers between the First and Second World Wars, but I refer to these three papers with a military theme because it was research into the experiences and behavioural problems of the Vietnam war veterans that produced the findings on which the American Psychiatric Association based their final definition of PTSD in the DSM. Further research was done after the Falklands conflict, and sadly there will doubtless be further research from the conflict in the Gulf.

How was it then that UK lawyers came to appreciate the relevance of non-physical injury following disaster? The 1985 Manchester air disaster helped to bring the issue into focus and my involvement with the victims's claims together with several years of representing patients suffering from mental disorder and membership of the Mental Health Act Commission meant that I had developed a special interest in this area. I had also been inspired by the speeches in the well-known decision of the House of Lords in *McLoughlin* v. *O'Brian* in 1982.[6] Mrs McLoughlin received compensation for nervous shock, even though she had not been present at the scene of the road accident which gravely injured her husband and children. To me, as a specialist personal injury and mental health lawyer, this was a fascinating development. A couple of years later I settled a case for a client on similar facts to Mrs McLoughlin, and through that process began to look more closely at compensation for traumatically induced psychiatric injury.

Then in 1985, when the Manchester air disaster happened, we retained American attorneys who helped us to negotiate what came to be known as a "mid-Atlantic settlement". From the Americans we learnt more about claims for what they call emotional distress, PTSD, and pre-impact terror. Since then these concepts have been considered and dealt with in different ways in each instant disaster that has happened in the UK. In two cases in particular, the *Herald of Free Enterprise* and the Hillsborough disaster, the courts have been involved. The most up-to-date assessment of the attitude of the courts towards the duty of care that must be breached before psychiatric injury is compensated is in the two judgments of Mr Justice Hidden in the Hillsborough case.[7] He considered 17 test cases brought by relatives who claimed compensation for psychiatric damage as a result of witnessing injuries to their loved ones, whether as eyewitnesses or by the means of communication by television or radio. In a comprehensive judgment, he reviewed the legal authorities on psychiatric injury coming from England, Canada and Australia, stating that "the law has evolved slowly over the last hundred years or so". A chronological summary of the cases he reviewed is as follows:

Psychiatric injury: the line of authorities

1886. *Victorian Railway Commissioners* v. *Coulta*[8] (Australia): No damages for nervous shock unaccompanied by physical injury.

1890. *Bell* v. *Great Northern Railway Co.*[9] Ireland: Damages awarded for nervous shock despite no physical injury.

1901. *Dulieu* v. *White*[10]: Damages awarded for nervous shock limited to fear for oneself only.

1925. *Hambrook* v. *Stokes*,[11]: Damages awarded for nervous shock apprehending fear for safety of children.

1932. *Donoghue* v. *Stevenson*[12]: Proximity does not merely mean physical proximity; it also extends to proximity of relationships between people.

1939. *Chester* v. *Waverley Corporation*[13] (Australia): No damages for nervous shock on seeing corpse of 7-year-old son – no duty of care.

1942. *Bourhill* v. *Young*[14]: The "pregnant fishwife". No damages for nervous shock on witnessing accident involving a stranger – no duty of care.

1953. *King* v. *Phillips*[15]: no damages for mother who heard screams of son and ran to scene – no duty of care.

1964. *Boardman* v. *Sanderson*[16]: Damages awarded to father who heard screams of son and ran to scene.

1967. *Abramzik* v. *Brenner*[17] (Canada): No damages to mother told of death of two children – no duty of care.

1868. *Dillon* v. *Legg*[18] (California: Damages awarded to mother for emotional shock and physical injury from witnessing death of her child.

1970. *Hinz* v. *Berry*[19]: Damages to mother witnessing accident to family.

The case of *Hinz* v. *Berry* is worthy of special mention because Lord Denning reviews the law, saying:

> The law at one time said that there could not be damages for nervous shock but for these last 25 years, it has been settled that damages can be given for nervous shock caused the sight of an accident at any rate to a close relative. . ./ In English law no damages are awarded for grief or sorrow caused by a person's death. No damages are to be given for worry about the children or for the financial strain or stress or the difficulties of adjusting to a new life. Damages are however recoverable for nervous shock or to put it in medical terms for any recognisable psychiatric illness caused by the breach of duty by the defendant.[20]

In this case Mrs Hinz, her husband and children were on a picnic by the roadside. Mrs Hinz was on one side of the road picking some flowers with one of the children. The rest of the family were on the other side of the road when a lorry ploughed into them. She witnessed the carnage that occurred.

> Somehow or other the Court has to draw a line between sorrow and grief for which damages are not recoverable and nervous shock and psychiatric illness for which damages are recoverable.

> The way to do this is to estimate how much Mrs Hinz would have suffered if for instance her husband had been killed in an accident when she was 50 miles away and compare it with what she is now, having suffered all the shock due to being present at the accident.[21]
>
> **AWARD £4000.**

One wonders how a judge can be expected to perform the intellectual gymnastics required to satisfy that test. As we proceed we will see how they have made attempts to do so.

1971. *Marshall* v. *Lionel Enterprises* (Canada)[22]: Damages awarded to wife for nervous shock when arriving on scene of accident to husband shortly afterwards.
1972. *Benson* v. *Lee* (Australia)[23]: Damages awarded to mother 100 yards away from accident to son on being told of it by other son and then running to scene.
1984. *McLoughlin* v. *O'Brian*:[24] Damages to wife and mother arriving at hospital afterwards and witnessing injuries to husband and children.
1984. *Janesch* v. *Coffey* (Australia)[25]: Damages to wife arriving at hospital afterwards and witnessing injuries to her husband.

In *Janesch* v. *Coffey*, Brennan J stated in the High Court of Australia that:

> Whether being told by friend or relative, in person or on the telephone, remains an open question.
>
> I understand "shock" in this context to mean the sudden sensory perception i.e. by seeing, hearing or touching of a person, thing or event which is so distressing that the perception of the phenomena affronts or insults the Plaintiff's mind and causes a psychiatric illness. A psychiatric illness induced by mere knowledge of a distressing fact is not compensable; perception by the Plaintiff of the distressing phenomena is essential[26].

Of the decisions since 1971 the case to discuss most extensively is *McLoughlin* v. *O'Brian* in 1982, a decision of the House of Lords. Mrs McLoughlin was telephoned at home and told of a terrible road accident to her husband and children, who were in a nearby hospital. An hour or so later she arrived to find her family being attended to in various states of severe injury. One of her three children had been killed. Understandably she was traumatised by the experience and claimed damages for her nervous shock. The vital point of the case is that Mrs McLoughlin was not at the scene of the accident but arrived at the hospital to see the aftermath. It was held that her proximity to the events and her relationship with those who had been injured were sufficiently close that she was entitled to compensation.

The last case in the sequence, *Attia* v. *British Gas*[27] is important because it deals with damages for nervous shock when Mrs Attia arrived home to find the emergency services present: her home had been blown up by a gas explosion and was on fire (the Gas Board had been trying to fit a new central heating system). The case is authority for the proposition that damages for psychiatric injury can include the traumatic event of seeing your home demolished. You may recall that in DSM III R the description of PTSD includes reference to damage to your home. The case is also a useful authority for the terminology to be used.

In *Attia* v. *British Gas* Bingham LJ stated:

> Her claim is accordingly one for what have in the authorities and the literature been called damages for nervous shock. Judges have in recent years become increasingly restive at the use of this misleading and inaccurate expression and I shall use the general expression "psychiatric damage" intending to comprehend within it all relevant forms of mental illness, neurosis and personality change. But the train of events (all of which must be causally related) with which this action like its predecessors is concerned remains unchanged. Careless conduct on the part of the Defendant causing actual or apprehended injury to the Plaintiff or a person other than the Defendant: the suffering of acute mental emotional trauma by the Plaintiff on witnessing or apprehending that injury or witnessing its aftermath: psychiatric damage suffered by the Plaintiff.[28]

Before I proceed to look more closely at the Hillsborough decision it is necessary to take a closer look at some of the speeches in *McLoughlin* v. *O'Brian.* I have selected relevant passages from the speeches of Lord Wilberforce and Lord Bridge where they cover much important ground as follows:

Lord Wilberforce said:

(a) On the subject of nervous shock:

> Although we continue to use the hallowed expression "nervous shock", English law and common understanding have moved

some distance since recognition was given to this symptom as a basis for liability. Whatever is unknown about the mind–body relationship (and the area of ignorance seems to expand with that of knowledge) it is now accepted by medical science that recognisable and severe physical damage to the human body and system may be caused by the impact through the senses of external events on the mind. There may thus be produced what is as identifiable an illness as any that may be caused by direct physical impact.[29]

(b) On the policy question of the extent of the legal parameters:

The policy arguments against a wider extension can be stated under four heads. First it may be said that such extension may lead to a proliferation of claims and possibly fraudulent claims, to the establishment of an industry of lawyers and psychiatrists who will formulate a claim for nervous shock damages including what in America is called the customary miscarriage for all or many, road accidents and industrial accidents. Secondly it may be claimed that extension of liability would be unfair to Defendants as imposing damages out of proportion to the negligent conduct complained of. Insofar as such Defendants are insured a large additional burden would be placed on insurers and ultimately upon the class of persons insured – road users or employers. Thirdly, to extend liability beyond the most direct and plain cases would greatly increase evidentiary difficulties and tend to lengthen litigation. Fourthly it may be said – and the Court of Appeal agreed with this – that an extension of the scope of liability ought only to be made by the legislature after careful research.[30]

(c) On the essential features of a claim by a person not at the scene:

It is necessary to consider three elements inherent in any claim: the class of persons whose claims should be recognised; the proximity of such persons to the accident; and the means by which the shock is caused. As regard the class of persons the possibility range is between the closest of family ties – of parent and child or husband and wife – and the ordinary bystander. Existing law recognises the claims of the first: it denies that of the second . . .

Lastly, as regards communication, there is no case in which the last has compensated shock brought by communication by a third party. The shock must come through sight or hearing of the event or of its immediate aftermath. Whether some equivalent of sight or hearing, e.g. through simultaneous television would suffice may have to be considered.[31]

Lord Bridge summed up neatly the medico-legal problem of assessing psychiatric injury:

> The basic difficulty of the subject arises from the fact that the crucial answers to the questions which it raises lie in the difficult field of psychiatric medicine. The common law gives no damages for the emotional distress which any normal person experiences when someone he loves is killed or injured. Anxiety and depression are normal human emotions. Yet an anxiety neurosis of a reactive depression may be recognisable psychiatric illnesses with or without psychosomatic symptoms. So the first hurdle which a Plaintiff claiming damages of the kind in question must surmount is to establish that he is suffering nor merely grief, distress or any other normal emotion but a positive psychiatric illness.[32]

In dealing with the court's traditionally cautious attitude towards psychiatric evidence Lord Bridge went on to say:

> For too long earlier generations of judges have regarded psychiatry and psychiatrists with suspicion if not hostility. Now I venture to hope that attitude has quite disappeared. No judge who has spent any length of time trying personal injury claims in recent years would doubt that physical injuries can give rise not only to organic but also to psychiatric disorders. The sufferings of the patient from the latter are no less real and frequently no less painful and disabling than the former. Likewise I would suppose that the legal profession well understands that an acute emotional trauma, like a physical trauma can well cause a psychiatric illness in a wide range of circumstances and in a wide range of individuals who it would be wrong to regard as having any abnormal psychological makeup. It is in comparatively recent times that these insights have come to be generally accepted by the Judiciary. It is only by giving effect to these insights and the developing law of negligence that we can do justice to an important though no doubt small class of Plaintiffs whose genuine psychiatric illnesses are caused by negligent defendants.[33]

It was the prophetic words of Lord Wilberforce referring to television which set the scene for the difficulties facing Mr Justice Hidden in the Hillsborough case.[34]

The Hillsborough case

The problems of proximity in time space and family relationship discussed in *McLoughlin* were tackled by Hidden J as he analysed that case:

> From the speeches of their Lordships in *McLoughlin* v. *O'Brian* it

> is clear that it is not only in the proximity of the relationship between the Plaintiff and the Victim of the accident that the common law must be free to move on, it is also in the degree of proximity in time and space to the accident and also the medium by which the shock deriving from the accident is communicated. But if the common law has the licence to move on with changing times then that licence must also be subject to a certain degree of limitation if the defendant who is guilty of some negligence is not to be made liable to the world at large. If the common law is entitled to extend the right to recovery for damages for nervous shock or rather psychiatric illness then one is forced to consider the three elements which are right for extension, namely:
>
> (i) the relationship between the Plaintiff and the original Victim of the Defendant's negligence – the loved one;
> (ii) the relationship in time and space between the Plaintiff and the scene of the original negligence;
> (iii) the medium through which the Plaintiff becomes conscious of the original negligence.[35]

Later, Hidden J continued:

> English law as we have seen permits only those within the relationship of spouse and parent to recover. The reasons for this are abundantly clear. It is only in cases where the relationship is of the closest known to man that it is reasonably foreseeable that the doing of physical harm to the one may cause mental harm amounting to true psychiatric illness to the other. It has until now been considered that in the spectrum of human relationships ranging from the closest of ties known to man through all degrees of relationship to that of the mere bystander it is only in the former in which it is reasonably foreseeable that such damage may follow. For all other relationships it is reasonably foreseeable that the possession of "reasonable phlegm" as the law puts it will prevent the onset of a psychiatric illness . . .
>
> I have to ask myself and then answer the question, ought that still to be the position in the light of modern knowledge and modern circumstances and in particular in the circumstances of this case? On the basis of where the line is at present drawn it is sensible first to consider the closest relationship which falls immediately outside that line, that of brother and sister. For a number of reasons I have concluded that, that line should include the brother or sister of the victim of negligence. I can see no basis in logic or in law why that relationship should be excluded.[36]

Having extended the proximity in relationship to brother and sister, Mr Justice Hidden excluded grandfather, uncle, fiancé, brother-in-law and friend.

In dealing with time and space and means of communication problems, it is worth pointing out that there were many relatives sitting at home in Liverpool watching live television. There were even some people, who couldn't get into the ground, who sat outside watching television in the coach. There were thus a number of different permutations of how people experienced their loved ones being injured and killed without actually being present themselves. In a penetrating analysis of a difficult problem Mr Justice Hidden concluded:

> I would venture to think it beyond per-adventure that the common law has moved on to the stage where it no longer requires in such cases presence at the scene of an accident and actual sight of it. The line has been moved to incorporate into the accident its immediate aftermath as defined and explained by Lord Wilberforce in *McLoughlin* v. *O'Brian*. If that be the case what guidance can that give in a world in which simultaneous television transmission of events into the living rooms of that world is now an every day event ... Thus, the television watcher in those circumstances is aware that he is augmenting his own eyesight by the lens of a camera in a distant position but that his eyes are receiving through the intervention of that camera lens images of what is actually happening as he sees them just as a store detective sees the goods being put in the pocket and not the basket although he is not physically present at the scene of the theft so it is that the television watcher sees the crowd surge forward in Pen 3 at the Leppings Lane end though he is not at Hillsborough ...
>
> It was reasonably foreseeable, as I find, that if unfortunate events took place which changed the event from a joyful sporting occasion to a tragic piece of disastrous news, cameras would or might be used to transmit those live pictures. It was also reasonably foreseeable that those live pictures would be seen by many of the nearest and dearest of those involved in the disaster. It was not merely foreseeable, it was a pound to a penny that on the afternoon of two FA Cup semi-finals in which Liverpool and Everton football clubs were both separately engaged the television sets of the city would have been switched on and eagerly watched for the latest news even though the matches themselves were not to be transmitted live. In those circumstances I find that all those who saw the disaster live on television do come within the line of proximity of time and space and I can therefore bring together the effect of my findings so far.[37]

It is the most relevant part of his comments.

The nine who won

Brian Harrison, 30, who watched from the west stand as the disaster developed, knowing that his two brothers were on the terraces below. Both died in the crush.

Steven Jones, 25, a student who watched live television as his brother died.

Mrs Maureen Mullaney, 39, who watched live television knowing that her two sons were there at the match. She learned hours later that both had been injured.

Mrs Karen Hankin, 30, a mother of two, whose husband died as she watched live television coverage.

Mrs Agnes Copoc, 56, and her husband Harold, 63, both watching live coverage as their son died.

Mrs Denise Hough, 31, who was watching live television as her brother died.

Robert Spearrit, 46, who watched live television. His brother was badly injured and his 14-year-old nephew died.

Mr William Pemberton, 58, who was in a coach outside the ground watching television as his son died.

Mrs Brenda Hennessey, 35, who saw live television coverage and lost her brother.

The six who lost

Mr John O'Dell, 42, who took his nephew to the match and sat in the stand as his nephew was on the terraces; the nephew was found safe. Claim failed because the family relationship was not close enough.

Mr Peter Coldicutt, 24, in the west stand as one of his friends was crushed and injured on the terraces. Action failed because of lack of family relationship.

Miss Alexandra Penk, 23, watched live television coverage as her fiancé died in the tragedy. Judge ruled relationship was not in law close enough.

Mr Joseph Kehoe, 59, whose 14-year-old grandson died. Action failed through lack of a close enough relationship and the fact that he heard disaster on radio and saw a recording but did not see it live on television.

Mr Robert Alcock, 52, whose brother-in-law died. Mr Alcock was in the stand, but family relationship held not to be close enough.

Miss Catherine Jones, 24, whose brother died. She heard of the disaster while out shopping and later heard radio coverage and saw recorded TV pictures. Claim failed because she did not see live coverage.

There was another aspect to the Hillsborough case relating to pre-death pain and suffering. These were claims by the administrators of three deceased, two of whom were sisters, for what was described as pre-death pain and suffering in the case of each plaintiff lasting for between 20 and 30 minutes. Counsel for the plaintiffs argued that all life must end in death and, paradoxically, a peaceful and painless death is itself an amenity of life. To be deprived of such a death and to be subject to a painful and terrifying death must be judged a very serious loss of amenity.

The Judge found this very difficult and in a separate judgment rejected this alleged type of damage saying:

> Even as I give this judgment I find myself struggling to resolve a conflict between two different emotions. Those emotions are present at the same time – sympathy and puzzlement. I have deep sympathy for Victoria and Sarah Hicks and for Colin Waifer and for their unhappy parents at the loss of young lives and probable ruination of older ones. But I have at the same time a degree of puzzlement as to how the law can even begin to assess the extent of the agony those young people went through in order to come to a figure of pounds and pence as legal compensation for pre-death suffering. I have a degree of doubt as to whether it is an exercise that the law should embark upon at all in circumstances such as these . . .
>
> Any parent, any person who has lost any loved one, wants to believe that the loss was as instantaneous as possible because of the love and affection they have had for that person. It is therefore in a sense anomalous that by bringing the claim which is brought in these cases they are forced into the position of arguing against that which they truly want to believe. It is again for this reason that I wonder if this is a route that the law should travel down in coming to its conclusions. The more I have sought to stand back from the emotion of the events the more I have concluded that where there has tragically been a death the exercise of seeking to separate pre-death pain and suffering from the fact of death is not one which the law is equipped to carry out at least in circumstances such as these when death is swift and sudden as shown by the medical evidence.[38]

The *Herald of Free Enterprise* arbitration

It is interesting that the failure of the pre-death pain and suffering argument contrasts with the *Herald of Free Enterprise* case, where the plaintiffs agreed with P & O a standard payment to the estate of each deceased of £5000 for pre-death pain and suffering. The *Herald* case also involved claims by relatives who experienced traumatic psychiatric injury, because, if you remember, the *Herald* capsize happened at about 7.30 on a Friday evening and there was a report on the 9 o'clock news that evening, together with a photograph of the ship. By the 10 o'clock news, and certainly by "Newsnight", there were live pictures on TV. In the same sense that there were live pictures of the Hillsborough disaster, the relatives of the *Herald* victims saw live TV coverage of the rescue. Nearly 70 relatives' claims have been brought in the *Herald* case but are unsolved pending the outcome of the Hillsborough appeals.

It is important to note that in the Hillsborough case the defendants accepted that all 16 plaintiffs (even those who lost) had actually suffered psychiatric injury. The argument was about proximity and relationship. As yet we do not know what damages have been paid for PTSD in Hillsborough. In the *Herald* case, however, there was a dispute with P & O about the proper level of damages for psychiatric injury. In some cases there was a dispute about whether a survivor had sustained psychiatric injury at all. Many of the survivors who had been on board became involved in a dispute as to the level of damages for the psychiatric injury they had suffered. Ten cases were selected to go to arbitration under a procedure laid down in the agreement that had earlier been reached with P & O. In February 1989 a panel of three QCs, chaired by Sir Michael Ogden, Michael Wright (now Mr Justice Wright) and William Crowther, heard a great deal of evidence from experts, including Professor Gunn and Professor Yale from the Institute of Psychiatry. The arbitrator's decision is not binding on the courts but has already proved persuasive in subsequent cases of psychiatric injury, whether or not sustained in a disaster. They decided seven main points of principle:

1. PTSD is a recognised psychiatric illness.
2. Many Zeebrugge victims suffered PTSD.
3. The DSM III R is a useful guide to diagnosis.
4. Pathological grief is a recognised psychiatric illness in excess

of normal grief.

5. Some survivors suffer from other psychiatric illnesses such as depression and it is possible to suffer from more than one psychiatric illness.
6. It may be reasonable for survivors to refuse to undergo treatment for psychiatric damage.
7. Account should be taken in individual cases of any vulnerability to future psychiatric illness.

They expanded their reasoning behind these seven findings as follows:

> *Nervous shock*: The respondents have conceded that all the claimants suffered nervous shock. This rather odd legal phrase does not connote shock in the sense in which it is often used in ordinary conversation. In *McLoughlin* v. *O'Brian* (1983) AC 410 at page 421 Lord Bridge said this of nervous shock:
>
>> "The basic difficulty of the subject arises from the fact that the crucial answers to the questions which it raises lie in the difficult field of psychiatric medicine. The common law gives no damages for the emotional distress which any normal person experiences when someone he loves is killed or injured. Anxiety and depression are normal human emotions. Yet an anxiety neurosis or a reactive depression may be recognizable psychiatric illness, with or without psychosomatic simptoms. So, the first hurdle which a plaintiff claiming damages of the kind in question must surmount is to establish that he is suffering, not merely grief, distress or any other normal emotion, but a positive psychiatric illness."
>
> *Post-traumatic stress disorder (PTSD)*: While the respondents conceded that all the claimants suffered from nervous shock, it was necessary for us to consider the nature of the illness from which each claimant suffered, mainly because identification of the nature of the illness enables conclusions to be drawn about prognosis in most cases.

The arbitrators' decision continued:

> Many of the Zeebrugge victims undoubtedly suffered from PTSD; of course, some victims suffered from some other psychiatric illness, e.g. depression at the same time. We are asked by the claimants to make a finding that DSM III R contains a suitable guide to diagnosis of PTSD. The reason for this request is that

> claims from other victims are outstanding and it is desired to use findings made in this Award when dealing with the outstanding cases. While we are anxious to be as helpful as possible to the parties, we do not feel able to be as dogmatic about this point as the claimants would wish us to be because points may arise in outstanding cases which have not arisen in this arbitration. Furthermore PTSD is a very recent concept and was revised in the 1987 edition of DSM III.
>
> *Pathological grief*: Amongst those who had been bereaved a common diagnosis was that of abnormal or pathological grief. It became common ground amongst the medical experts that the circumstances of a bereavement could be significant in determining whether the subsequent grief would be pathological or normal and that a person who lost a relative in horrific circumstances was more likely to suffer from pathological grief than if the relative had died in more normal circumstances.

The arbitrators' decision continued:

> Some of the claimants lost one or more relatives in the disaster and suffered from what is termed "pathological grief" or "pathological mourning". This, too, is a recognised psychiatric illness and in non-medical terms can be said to be grief the extent and duration of which is in excess of normal grief reaction.
>
> This has posed extremely difficult problems of an obvious nature. As Lord Bridge said in the passage already quoted, a person is not to be compensated for normal grief. However, a person is to be compensated for pathological grief. "Normal" grief varies widely between one individual and another. Gauging the extent to which a claimant's suffering from grief which that claimant would have suffered is a task which is enormously difficult and cannot be undertaken with any degree of precision. In each case, we have had to estimate the extent to which the claimant's grief is in excess of the normal grief which the claimant would have suffered had the death occurred in ordinary circumstances and compensate the claimant accordingly. Obviously this can be done only in a very rough and ready fashion; the more so since in all these cases there is another form of illness present.

The arbitrators considered the question of prognosis as follows:

> *The duration of the illness*: Unhappily some of the claimants continue to suffer to a significant degree. However, in all cases improvement is probable and, in most, complete recovery is probable. This is not to say that the victim will ever forget the experience or that painful intrusive thoughts will cease. Plainly, that it impossible.

However, in such cases the improvement will reach a point at which it can be said that in spite of remaining intrusive thoughts etc., the victim is no longer suffering from psychiatric illness. Since compensation for nervous shock is compensation for psychiatric illness, it is the period until illness ceases which is compensatable. This has to be assessed, as has everything else, on a balance of probabilities and, for obvious reasons, the estimate approaches being the useful but nasty word "guesstimate".

However, in reaching our conclusions, we have borne in mind that most if not all prognoses are guarded in cases in which a claimant is still ill. Counsel for the claimant has urged us to bear in mind that, quite apart from the guarded nature of the prognosis, very understandably some claimants are reluctant to undergo treatment which involves recollecting the distressing circumstances of the disaster and may balk at undergoing such treatment. We have no hesitation in accepting this argument.

The arbitrators also considered the risk of future problems.

Vulnerability: An injury to a limb leaves it vulnerable. It is the same with psychiatric problems. All the claimants will be at risk of further illness in the face of stress which would not have affected them or would have affected them less but for the Zeebrugge experience. This is a factor which must be taken into account when assessing compensation. Following a serious head injury, there is often a risk of epilepsy and an award of damages takes account of that risk. Our awards do likewise in respect of vulnerability to future psychiatric troubles. In our view, it is an important factor which must be borne in mind in each case, although more so in some cases than in others.

In considering their awards of damages the arbitrators said:

Assessment of Damages: In 1970, in *Hinz* v. *Berry* [1970] 2 QB 40, Lord Denning MR said there were only two cases in which the quantum of damages for nervous shock had been considered and Lord Pearson said that he thought it was the first case in which the Court of Appeal had considered the problem.

Although counsel have gone to great trouble in assembling a comprehensive list of reported cases of damages for nervous shock, the number of such cases is comparatively small. More important, counsel agreed that no clear guidelines can be discerned in the reported cases.

In these circumstances, our assessment must be based not only upon consideration of the cases to which our attention was directed but also upon consideration of how each claimant's illness compares with cases in which damages were awarded for physical injuries.

In undertaking this task, we must record our appreciation for the very considerable help given to us by the doctors who gave evidence. It was fortunate both for us and the parties that, plainly, they are of the very highest calibre and competence.

In the ten following cases which were considered by the arbitrators, an asterisk represents the amount actually awarded by the arbitrators; all other amounts were either agreed amounts or the fixed payment noted earlier.

Case "A"

A 22-year-old single woman with some pre-existing fear of water. Civil servant. All her party survived. After 24 hours, reaction set in and she wept uncontrollably for two or three days. For several months she had a fear of water so intense that she could not take a bath without someone present to encourage her. She suffered PTSD for about nine months, with nightmares, loss of appetite, loss of libido, feelings of guilt and intrusive thoughts about the capsize. She constantly relived the accident in her mind. In July 1987 psychotherapy was recommended but not taken up. While her fear of water led her to cancel a trip to Sweden in 1987, in 1988 she was able to fly to Corfu and enjoy her holiday although she did not swim. She had received no treatment. The arbitrators found that for practical purposes she had entirely recovered by September 1988. Her physical injuries included bruising to her chest, back, right leg, arm, hands and left index finger. At the site of the bruising on her leg she had developed an irritable skin condition although with treatment the prognosis was good.

Total compensation of £9135.75 was made up as follows:

Fixed payment	£5000.00	
Psychiatric injuries	£1750.00*	
Physical injuries	£1250.00	
Special damages	£1135.75	
	£9135.75	plus interest to be calculated.

There was no award for loss of future earnings/earning capacity.

Case "B"

A 41-year-old married woman. All her party survived. By nine months post-accident she described symptoms of PTSD which were said by the medical experts to be moderately severe and she was said to be moderately depressed and anxious. She was described as "cheerful and coping" by November 1988 and had been able to resume work as a cashier. Her principal persistent symptom was an unwillingness to be parted from her husband even for short periods, to such an extent that she had obtained work at the same place as him. However, treatment was advised and the arbitrators found that with treatment she should be back to normal within about 12 months. She had sustained lacerations of her left hand with damage to the tendons in the ring and little fingers and to the digital nerves, ruptured ligaments of the left thumb and multiple contusions including a probable contusion of the right kidney. The left wrist and thumb were in plaster for three weeks and in August 1987 she underwent tendon graft under general anaesthetic when her hand was put in plaster for 12 weeks. She was left with some slight scarring disability and restriction of movement in the hand.

Total compensation of £20 160.82 was made up as follows:

Fixed payment	£5 000.00	
Psychiatric injuries	£3 000.00	
Cost of treatment for psychiatric injuries	£750.00	
Physical injuries	£8 250.00	
Special damages	£3 160.82	
	£20 160.82	plus interest to be calculated.

There was no award for loss of future earnings/earning capacity.

Case "C"

A 22-year-old single man. He and his travelling companion both survived. He was employed as a recreation assistant at swimming baths and was hoping to progress to a career in recreational management. He suffered from quite severe PTSD in the months immediately after the incident and consumption of alcohol increased substantially. By November 1988 the symptoms were said to be of moderate severity and consumption of alcohol had reverted to pre-accident level. The arbitrators approached the case on the basis that it was one of moderate psychiatric damage lasting for about 3.5 years. He had to give up his job, which he greatly enjoyed, and was now a chauffeur for a car hire firm which gave him very little job satisfaction. The arbitrators took into account that at present he was not suffering any loss of earnings or loss of leisure because he was working about the same hours as before and earning slightly more but he had lost his chance of promotion within his chosen career, which would have brought higher earnings for shorter hours. The arbitrators thought it likely, however, that once his psychiatric symptoms had abated he would find more congenial and remunerative employment. He had no physical injuries.

Total compensation of £21 728.30 was made up as follows:

Fixed payment	£5 000.00	
Psychiatric injuries	£4 000.00*	
Loss of chance of increased leisure/ potential loss of earnings	£2 000.00*	
Actual loss of earnings	£7 309.84	
Special damages	£3 418.46	
	£21 728.30	plus interest to be calculated.

There was no award for loss of future earnings/earning capacity.

Case "D"

A long-distance lorry driver travelling alone, married and aged 42. He suffered severe PTSD involving anxiety, sleeplessness and nightmares, sweating attacks and phobias of water and the sea. The sight of plate-glass windows or the sound of children crying caused him to think of the capsize. He had become severely depressed, irritable and aggressive. In the early stages he was drinking to excess but this problem had now been resolved. His level of smoking had also greatly increased and remained high. He found his work as a long-distance driver distressing because it meant he was on his own for a great deal of the time and on such occasions his mind dwelt on the capsize. He had therefore changed to work within the depot. It is highly unlikely that he will ever return to his old job. Because of his condition his marriage had come under serious strain. The doctors agreed that he would benefit from a period of regular psychiatric help for his anxiety states, coupled with specific treatment for depression. Although he was naturally resistant to such treatment the arbitrators found that with the support of his wife he would undergo treatment and that over the next 12–18 months he is likely to make a substantial improvement. Everyone accepted that over the last two years his illness had operated at a very severe level and had greatly exacerbated his vulnerability to stress for the foreseeable future. He had also suffered bruising and whilst acting as a rescuer in the capsize he had strained both his shoulders as a result of hauling on ropes. These had caused significant discomfort for some three months and he is still having some features of painful arc syndrome in his right shoulder. He had also strained both wrists and suffered some discomfort in his back.

Total compensation of £21 580.00 was made up as follows:

Fixed payment	£5 000.00	
Psychiatric injuries	£8 500.00*	
Physical injuries	£2 500.00	
Special damages	£580.00	
A loss of future earnings/earning capacity	£5 000.00**	
	£21 580.00	plus interest to be calculated.

**This was awarded because the arbitrators accepted that he now had to work longer and harder hours in less congenial employment to maintain his former level of earnings and that if he should give up or lose his present job his range of possible jobs would be restricted because he could not return to long-distance driving, but that suitable alternative work could be found by his employers, who were a large organisation.

Case "E"

A 38-year-old divorced woman with a teenage daughter (who was also a survivor) living at home. She had been travelling with her mother, to whom she was very close, and who was killed in dramatic circumstances. The mother's body was not recovered until it was washed ashore some three weeks after the capsize. There was a difference of opinion between the doctors whether she was suffering from an abnormal grief reaction or from hysterical dissociation as a defensive mechanism. It was accepted that either she was suffering from or would suffer from pathological grief and that hysterical dissociation, if present, was designed to protect her feelings of unusually severe grief. She took a great deal of time off work, and had counselling sessions and some in-patient treatment. In addition to her grief reactions she was still suffering from classic and severe PTSD, which has been unremitting since the accident, and depression, which had greatly improved so as no longer to be pathological. She was hoping to move home soon, in which event the prognosis was that within a further year from the move she would be back at work. She would need regular counselling and treatment for depression as an outpatient for one year. She is always likely to be vulnerable to stress but she had very considerable job security as a civil servant, so that the likelihood of her losing her job was remote in the extreme. In addition she had suffered generalised cuts and bruising.

Total compensation of £30 774.07 was made up as follows:

Fixed payment	£5 000.00	
Psychiatric injuries	£7 500.00*	
Cost of future treatment for psychiatric injuries	£1 000.00*	
Physical injuries	£400.00	
Loss of earnings to date	£4 398.89	
Future loss of earnings	£4 463.43*	
Fixed payment for loss of relative	£5 000.00	
Special damages	£3 011.75	
	£30 774.07	plus interest to be calculated.

Case "F"

A married man aged 41 years. His wife and two friends were killed in the capsize. He had developed chronic PTSD. In particular he was hypersensitive to unexpected noises and suffered panic attacks when faced with reminders of the capsize such as a 10-minute boat trip. His sleep was frequently disturbed and he had become irritable and impatient. He had suffered a profound pathological grief reaction. The arbitrators found that every aspect of his everyday life has been affected by the fact that she (his wife) is no longer with him. There was a discount in respect of the grief which he would have suffered if his wife had died in more ordinary circumstances. He was having difficulties with concentration and was thus afraid about the loss of his job in a managerial position. Outpatient treatment was recommended for 12–18 months, after which he should have achieved a substantial degree of recovery. He would remain vulnerable to stressful incidents for the foreseeable future. By way of physical injuries he suffered a chest infection which required hospital treatment, multiple bruises and grazes, local numbness in both heels and discomfort in the right shin. He had also suffered 10% loss of hearing in the left ear and tinnitus due to vascular damage as a result of stress. This had been diagnosed as Ménière's disease, giving rise to a 10% risk of bilateral hearing loss. A "tullio" phenomenon had also been diagnosed, which is a startle reaction to veer off (in this case to the right-hand side) on hearing a loud noise. He had also suffered some vertigo.

Total compensation (which does not include the fatal accident claim in respect of his wife's death) of £41 042.94 was made up as follows:

Fixed payment	£5 000.00	
Psychiatric injuries	£7 500.00*	
Cost of treatment for psychiatric injuries	£1 000.00	
Physical injuries	£20 000.00	
Further fixed payment for loss of relative	£5 000.00	
Special damages	£2 542.94	
	£41 042.94	plus interest to be calculated.

The arbitrators made no award for loss of earning capacity on the basis that he had managed to continue working in a sophisticated and highly competitive environment during the period since the capsize and was not under any real disadvantage in respect of his earning capacity.

Case "G"

A divorced lady aged 31 who had been living with a man for some three years before the capsize in which he was killed. His body was not recovered until the vessel was righted on 7 April 1987. She was said to have been one of the most severely affected of the survivors with whom the doctors had been concerned, and to have had a terrible two years. She was subject to mood swings, being tearful, miserable and very depressed, with suicidal thoughts, and she had been drinking to excess. She had become withdrawn and isolated from her friends, was very reckless about her own safety and was found to be suffering from a severe depressive illness. She had occasional outpatient sessions with a psychiatrist, which had not produced much improvement. She needs intensive supportive psychotherapy on a weekly basis for at least 12 months, in which case there was a reasonable prospect of getting her on her feet within 18 months from the arbitration. She would quite possibly find herself in stressful situations in the future and being sensitised to further disaster might well have serious problems in the future, however successful the short-term treatment may be. The arbitrators found her to be one of the claimants most vulnerable to further problems both in the near and more distant future. She had been in responsible and taxing work as an international auditor, which she had to give up. She was now hoping to start a small business. If all went well she would in about 4.5 years be back to earning as much as she would have earned but for the accident. Her actual loss over that period would be £36 000 but there was a real risk that because of her psychiatric condition the business would fail, which would cause both psychiatric and financial problems. The arbitrators held that they had to make appropriate allowance for the very substantial risk of unforeseen difficulties. She had also suffered bruising around her midriff and on the legs.

Total compensation (which did not include the fatal accident claim in respect of her co-habitee) £98 333.00 was made up as follows:

Fixed payment	£5 000.00	
Psychiatric injuries	£15 000.00*	
Physical injuries	£400.00	
Loss of earnings to date	£21 557.00	
Loss of future earnings/earning capacity	£50 000.00	
Fixed payment for loss of relative	£5 000.00	
Special damages	£1 376.00	
	£98 333.00	plus interest to be calculated.

Case "H"

An 11-year-old boy travelling with his family. His mother and elder brother were killed. His father and sister survived. In September 1987 he was diagnosed as suffering from chronic PTSD and prolonged depressive adjustment reaction. By June 1988 he was severely depressed and at times suicidal. His schooling was disrupted by non-attendance. He was still depressed and suffering from PTSD at the time of the arbitration and the arbitrators found him to be severely disturbed. The prognosis was quite good in that with proper inpatient treatment for five to six weeks with continuing outpatient care he would be on his feet in 18 months to two years. The arbitrators hoped for a very substantial recovery but found a significant risk that treatment would not be successful and he would still be vulnerable to relapse. Before the capsize the claimant was probably of "A" level ability and might with very hard work have obtained university entrance. With treatment he was expected to return to full-time education but there was a significant risk that he would not and would therefore have no academic qualifications. Even if he went back to his studies and recovered most of his pre-accident potential he would be a late starter with a good deal of catching up to do. He would be permanently vulnerable to stress and would have to avoid jobs of a particularly stressful nature. Even if he avoided such jobs he would be vulnerable to relapse and consequent periods of unemployment. He suffered the following physical injuries:

1. Avulsion of the transverse processes from his first, second, third and fourth lumbar vertebrae on the right side. There was acute pain initially which subsided after about one month and thereafter continued at a reduced level for a further two months or so. He continues to have pain on stressing his back but the prognosis is good. However, it is unlikely that transverse processes will fuse again at their fracture site, which could create problems if he has to do a lot of lifting. His earning capacity is thus further impaired. He has been advised against participating in sports such as athletics, rugby or football. There will be permanent disability as he will tend to get aching in his lumbar spine particularly after heavy use.
2. Severe bruising in the area of the kidneys. He had an intravenous urogram to which he had an allergic reaction such that he almost died.

3. A urinary tract infection.
4. He developed eczema of both hands and thighs and it is likely that stress following the disaster has been a factor in producing the disorder. Although there has been improvement, prognosis is uncertain.
5. Generalised cuts and bruises.

Total compensation of £102 453.00 was made up as follows:

Fixed payment	£5 000.00	
Psychiatric injuries	£20 000.00*	
Cost of treatment for psychiatric injuries	£8 000.00	
Physical injuries	£7 500.00	
Future loss of earnings/earning capacity	£50 000.00*	
Fixed payments for loss of relatives	£10 000.00	
Special damages	£1 953.00	
	£102 453.00	plus interest to be calculated.

Case "I"

A married man aged 26 whose wife and 4-month old daughter were travelling with him. He and the baby survived but his wife was killed. He was an enlisted soldier but was discharged in July 1988 as no longer medically fit for service. He had formed an intense relationship with his wife and the army. Having lost both he was now on his own and totally lost. He drinks and smokes heavily. By December 1988 he was still profoundly depressed, with a high level of anxiety and intrusive obsessional thoughts. With treatment, recovery would take at least another two years and this was optimistic. He was, however, extremely resistant to treatment, which was symptomatic of his condition. Without successful treatment and without regaining some motivation in life the outlook was gloomy. With successful treatment he will have four to five years of severe disability. He had suffered a contusion of the chest and two fractured ribs, with some contusion of the underlying lung and one episode of haemoptysis (coughing blood). He continues to experience aching in his chest when carrying out heavy work or during inclement weather.

Total compensation (excluding fatal accident claim in respect of his wife) of £148 571.12 was made up as follows:

Fixed payment	£5 000.00
Psychiatric injuries	£15 000.00*
Physical injuries	£2 250.00
Loss of earnings to date	£8 000.00
Loss of future earnings/earning capacity/army pension rights	£109 500.00
Fixed payment for loss of relative	£5 000.00
Special damages	£3 821.12
	£148 571.12 plus interest to be calculated.

Case "J"

A 54-year-old married man working as a tractor driver at a main-line railway terminal. His mother, wife, daughter and 10-month-old grandchild (all of whom had lived in the same household with him) were killed. The emotional and psychological impact of the disaster had been catastrophic. He is suffering from a depressive illness, pathological grief and severe PTSD. He had suicidal thoughts and had become a heavy drinker and smoker. He was receiving inpatient treatment at the time of the arbitration. The arbitrators found him to be demoralised, bitterly unhappy and depressed and at present totally unable to reconstruct his life. He would never be able to work again. The prognosis was extremely gloomy. Over a period of up to five years with treatment he may become more comfortable with his daily life and may be able to take up some hobby or interest to occupy his mind. His present grief, depression and anxiety would always be with him to some extent. He was the worst of all the survivors the doctors had seen. He was suffering from a pathological grief reaction but the arbitrators bore in mind that anyone who suffered the loss of four relatives would be likely to suffer considerable grief and that they had to assess the extent to which his reaction exceeded that which would be expected after the death of four relatives in other circumstances. He also suffered a hand injury, a whiplash injury of the cervical spine, an injury to the right elbow and an injury to the right middle finger. He has some continuing discomfort in his neck. His right elbow is stiff and will not straighten properly and he has intermittent triggering of the right finger. He has difficulty lifting weights such as suitcases, and stretching up and doing DIY jobs.

Total compensation (excluding fatal accident claims for deceased relatives) of £151 114.27 was made up as follows:

Fixed payment	£5 000.00	
Psychiatric injuries	£30 000.00*	
Physical injuries	£5 500.00*	
Loss of earnings to date	£19 026.00	
Future loss of earnings	£65 880.00*	
Cost of DIY	£2 000.00	
Fixed payments for lost relative	£20 000.00	
Special damages	£3 708.27	
	£151 114.27	plus interest to be calculated.

Some concluding remarks

Finally, I should consider the question of "legal trauma", which in itself is an increasingly large subject. There has been a good deal of public debate in the aftermath of disaster regarding, particularly, "corporate responsibility". It is my belief that the sequence of procedures in the aftermath of recent disasters has been so varied that there is no discernible pattern that could even be described as a system that victims or the public can understand. I suggest that there is a pressing need for a system that gives access to one speedy and thorough inquiry into all the relevant issues. The number and nature of inquiries that may come into operation at present vary according to the nature of the disaster. The possibilities include a public inquiry initiated by the Minister on criteria that are obscure, an internal inquiry, an inquiry and report to the Minister by the Aviation Investigation Branch or the Maritime Accident Investigation Branch, or a British Rail inquiry, or an inquest and/or criminal investigation that may or may not lead to prosecution. Any combination of these inquiries is likely to create undesirable procedural problems that may inhibit the efficient disposal of the post-disaster issues; I will briefly indicate what I think they are.

In my view, following a disaster, there are five things to which the survivors, bereaved relatives and the public want to know answers:

1. how it happened;
2. how each deceased met his or her death;
3. how the disaster could have been avoided;
4. safety;
5. assessment and apportionment of blame.

The present system makes it difficult for those five questions to be addressed in a sensible sequence of answers.

The need for reform is illustrated by some of the problems of the victims and families in the *Marchioness* disaster, a case which has posed Dr Knapman, HM Coroner for Westminster, some difficulties over the inquest. Eighteen months after the disaster the victims still await a full explanation of what happened and why it happened. They have had no access to a full public inquiry. The decision by the Director of Public Prosecutions to prosecute the captain of the *Bowbelle* has impeded the publication of the full Maritime Accident Investigation Branch report and prevented Dr Knapman from holding a full inquest. An application for judicial review of the limited scope of the prosecution was unsuccessful. Mr Justice Nolan gave some consoling remarks when he said in his judgment:"The sinking of the *Marchioness* was an appalling tragedy. It is entirely understandable that the survivors and relatives of those who died and those concerned with the safe passage of vessels on the Thames seek a full public inquiry into its causes. The Secretary of State for Transport remained steadfast in his refusal to announce a public inquiry.

Following a disaster there is a difficult interface between the findings of a public inquiry, the recommendations of a report by the Accident Investigation Branch, the inquest verdict of a jury and the outcome of a criminal prosecution. In whatever sequence they are held these different inquiries may produce incongruous results that bewilder the public, particularly in the example where an unlawful killing verdict by a jury does not result in a criminal conviction trial.

The corporate responsibility debate, fuelled by the collapse of the *Herald* trial and the contrasting jailing of the Purley train driver, will continue, but represents only one aspect of a wider problem. A letter to *The Times* in October suggested the appointment of a Royal Commission headed by a High Court Judge. However, recent history suggests that the government is firmly set against the use of Royal Commissions, because they take too long to assess and report, and although the need for reform is urgent, the range of issues that require attention, in my view, is insufficiently wide to justify a Royal Commission.

Another idea circulating at the moment is the formation of a small working party with a limited remit and a short period to consult and report. Many people are not aware of the fact that the Home Secretary has a Civil Emergencies Adviser, retired Air Commodore David Brooke, whose remit gives him an important voice in these matters. An equally important voice is that of the victims themselves, who have recently formed a group known as Disaster Action as a conglomerate of a number of the action groups of various disasters.

I would suggest that immediately after every disaster a High Court judge should be appointed to conduct an inquiry in public into how, when, where and why the disaster occurred and how any fatalities occurred. The judge would have wide powers, including those of a coroner, or could sit with a coroner (perhaps even better) and would also sit, if necessary with professional assessors. The evidence for the inquiry would be gathered by the police, working in conjunction with whichever agency has the relevant technical expertise, such as the Maritime Branch in a maritime case. The judge would have powers to supervise and ensure that the evidence is gathered swiftly and efficiently. To complete the picture and to recognise public concern for the corporate responsibility factor if it is a feature, it would be necessary to give the judge power to reflect judicial disapproval of reckless or grossly negligent behaviour by the imposition of a fine, if necessary of swingeing proportions. Such a fine could go towards the cost of research and development of the emergency services' response to disasters or into pre-disaster contingency planning and post-disaster response.

The early judicial oversight of the civil aspects of compensation in complex group actions is now well established in what I referred to earlier as "the creeping disasters". In the Opren, HIV-positive haemophiliacs and benzodiazepine litigations, the courts intervened at an early stage to provide judicial oversight. It would be consistent to extend this trend to the aftermath of transport and other instant disasters. Problems will still exist so I do not suggest this as a panacea, but it is a starting point by which I believe the legal trauma to the victims will be much reduced.

Appendix 1: DSM III R 309.89 Post-traumatic Stress Disorder

The essential feature of this disorder is the development of characteristic symptoms following a psychologically distressing event that is outside the range of usual human experience (i.e. outside the range of such common experiences as simple bereavement, chronic illness, business losses, and marital conflict). The stressor producing this syndrome would be markedly distressing to almost anyone, and is usually experienced with intense fear, terror, and helplessness. The characteristic symptoms involve re-experiencing the traumatic event, avoidance of stimuli associated with the event of numbing of general responsiveness, and increased arousal. The diagnosis is not made if the disturbance lasts less than one month.

The most common traumata involve either a serious threat to one's life or physical integrity; a serious threat or harm to one's children, spouse, or other close relatives and friends; sudden destruction of one's home or community; or seeing another person who has recently been, or is being seriously injured or killed as the result of an accident or physical violence. In some cases the trauma may be learning about a serious threat or harm to a close friend or relative, e.g. that one's child has been kidnapped, tortured or killed.

The traumatic event can be re-experienced in a variety of ways. Commonly the person has recurrent and intrusive recollections of the event or recurrent distressing dreams during which the event is re-experienced. In rare instances there are dissociative states, lasting from a few seconds to several hours, or even days, during which components of the event are re-lived, and the person behaves as though experiencing the event at that moment. There is often intense psychological distress when the person is exposed to events that resemble an aspect of the traumatic event or that symbolize the traumatic event, such as anniversaries of the event.

In addition to the re-experiencing of the trauma, there is persistent avoidance of stimuli associated with it, or a numbing of general responsiveness that was not present before the trauma. The person commonly makes deliberate efforts to avoid thoughts or feelings about the traumatic event and about activities or situations that arouse recollections of it. This avoidance of reminders of the trauma may include psychogenic amnesia for an important aspect of the traumatic event.

Diminished responsiveness to the external world, referred to as "psychic numbing" or "emotional anaesthesia", usually begins soon after the traumatic event. A person may complain of feeling detached or estranged from other people, that he or she has lost the ability to become interested in previously enjoyed activities, or that ability to feel emotions of any type, especially those associated with intimacy, tenderness, and sexuality, is markedly decreased.

Persistent symptoms of increased arousal that were not present before the trauma include difficulty falling or staying asleep (recurrent nightmares during which the traumatic event is re-lived are sometimes accompanied by middle or terminal sleep disturbance), hypervigilance, and exaggerated startle response. Some complain of difficulty in concentrating or in completing tasks. Many report changes in aggression. In mild cases this may take the form of irritability with fears of losing control. In more severe forms, particularly in cases in which the survivor has actually committed acts of violence (as in war veterans), the fear is conscious and pervasive, and the reduced capacity for modulation may express itself in unpredictable or aggressive behaviour or an inability to express angry feelings.

Associated features: symptoms of depression and anxiety are common, and in some instances may be sufficiently severe to be diagnosed as an Anxiety or Depressive Disorder. Impulsive behaviour can occur, such as suddenly changing place of residence, unexplained absence, or other changes in life-style. There may be symptoms of an Organic Mental Disorder, such as failing memory, difficulty in concentrating, emotional lability, headache, and vertigo. In the case of a life-threatening trauma shared with others, survivors often describe painful guilt feelings about surviving when others did not, or about the things they had to do in order to survive.

Appendix 2: diagnostic criteria for 309.89 Post-traumatic Stress Disorder

It also lists the diagnostic criteria as follows:

A. The person has experienced an event that is outside the range of usual human experience and that would be markedly distressing to anyone, e.g. serious threat to one's life or physical integrity; serious threat or harm to one's children, spouse, or other close relative and friends; sudden destruction of one's home or community; or seeing another person who has recently been, or is being seriously injured or killed as the result of an accident or physical violence.

B. The traumatic event is persistently re-experienced in at least one of the following ways:

(1) recurrent and intrusive distressing recollections of the

event (in young children, repetitive play in which themes or aspects of the trauma are expressed);
(2) recurrent distressing dreams of the event;
(3) sudden acting or feeling as if the traumatic event were recurring (includes a sense of re-living the experience, illusions, hallucinations, and dissociative [flashback] episodes, even those that occur upon awakening or when intoxicated);
(4) intense psychological distress at exposure to events that symbolize or resemble an aspect of the traumatic event, including anniversaries of the trauma.

C. Persistent avoidance of stimuli associated with the trauma or numbing of general responsiveness (not present before the trauma) as indicated by at least three of the following:
(1) efforts to avoid thoughts or feelings associated with the trauma:
(2) efforts to avoid activities or situations that arouse recollections of the trauma;
(3) inability to recall an important aspect of the trauma (psychogenic amnesia);
(4) markedly diminished interest in significant activities (in young children, loss of recently acquired developmental skills such as toilet training or language skills);
(5) feeling of detachment or estrangement from others;
(6) restricted range of affect, e.g. unable to have loving feelings;
(7) sense of foreshortened future, e.g. does not extend to have a career, marriage or children or a long life.

D. Persistent symptoms of increased arousal (not present before the trauma), as indicated by at least two of the following:
(1) difficulty falling or staying asleep;
(2) irritability or outbursts of anger;
(3) difficulty concentrating;
(4) hypervigilance;
(5) exaggerated startle response;
(6) physiological reactivity upon exposure to events that symbolize or resemble an aspect of the traumatic event (e.g. a woman who was raped in an elevator breaks out in a sweat when entering any elevator).

E. Duration for the disturbance (symptoms in B, C and D) of at least one month).

Notes and References

1. Pannone, "Forum shopping: trans-national claims" (1987) 55 *Medico-Legal Journal* 224.
2. *Attia* v. *British Gas plc* [1987] 3 All ER 455 at 462 per Bingham LJ.

3. (1917) *British Medical Journal* 39.
4. (1943) *British Medical Journal* 703 and 740.
5. Swank, "Combat Exhaustion" [1949] 109 *Journal of Nervous & Mental Diseases* 475.
6. [1982] 2 All ER 298.
7. [1991] 1 All ER 353.
8. (1888) 13 App. Cas. 222.
9. (1890) 26 LR Ir. 328.
10. [1901] 2 KB 669.
11. [1925] 1 KB 141.
12. [1932] AC 562.
13. (1939) 62 CLR 1.
14. [1943] AC 92.
15. [1953] 1 QB 429.
16. [1964] 1 WLR 1317.
17. (1967) 65 DLR (2d) 65l.
18. (1968) 441 P 2d 912.
19. [1970] 2 QB 40.
20. Ibid at 42.
21. Ibid at 43.
22. [1972] 2 OR 177.
23. [1972] VR 879.
24. [1982] 2 All ER 298.
25. (1984) 54 ALR 417.
26. Ibid at 462.
27. [1987] 3 All ER 455.
28. Ibid at 462.
29. Supra note 6 at 301.
30. Ibid at 303–4.
31. Ibid at 304–5.
32. Ibid at 311.
33. Ibid at 312–3.
34. *Jones* v. *Wright* [1991] 1 All ER 353.
35. Ibid at 371.
36. Ibid at 375.
37. Ibid at 378–81.
38. (*Unreported.*) The Court of Appeal and House of Lords dismissed the plaintiff's appeal: *Hicks* v. *Chief Constable of South Yorkshire Police* [1992] 1 All ER 690 and [1992] 2 All ER 65.

Editor's note

On appeal in the Hillsborough case, the Court of Appeal [1991] 3 All ER 88) and subsequently, the House of Lords in *Alcock* v. *Chief Constable of South Yorkshire Police* [1991] 4 All ER 907) held that the plaintiffs' claims failed. First, the House of Lords held that a claim for nervous shock or psychiatric injury required a plaintiff to establish a close relationship of love and affection with the injured or dead victims. Such a relationship would be presumed between parent and child, spouses or an engaged couple, but had to be established by evidence in all other relationships, for example, between brothers, brothers-in-law or grandfather and grandson. On this basis, all but two of the plaintiffs failed since no evidence had been presented to the trial judge to establish the closeness of their relationships with the victims. Secondly, the House of Lords held that a claim could only succeed if a plaintiff was at the scene of the disaster or its immediate aftermath. However, viewing the scene on television (whether live or otherwise) or hearing of the events on the radio was not equivalent to this, nor was identifying a victim's body at the mortuary sufficient. On this basis, the claims of the remaining plaintiffs, whose son and fiancé had died, failed.

The decision of the House of Lords has implications for psychiatric injury claims arising from facts not in issue in *Alcock*, for example, where the plaintiff is told of the relative's death (*Ravenscroft* v. *Rederiaktiebolaget Transatlantic* (note) [1992] 2 All ER 470).

For a discussion of the case and its wider implications see Lunney, "Hillsborough: the one that got away (1992) 3 *King's College Law Journal* 170.

Index

Choices and Decisions in Health Care. Edited by A. Grubb.

Index compiled by Campbell Purton